Qi Energy

for Health and Healing

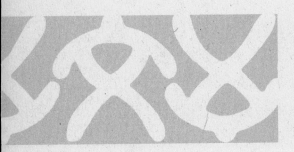

Qi Energy

AVERY

A MEMBER OF PENGUIN GROUP (USA) INC.

NEW YORK

Qi Energy
for Health and Healing

A COMPREHENSIVE GUIDE TO
ACCESSING YOUR HEALING ENERGY

MALLORY FROMM, Ph.D.

ILLUSTRATIONS BY PAMELA HARTMAN

Most Avery books are available at special quantity discounts for bulk purchase for sales promotions, premiums, fund-raising, and educational needs. Special books or book excerpts also can be created to fit specific needs. For details, write Penguin Group (USA) Inc. Special Markets, 375 Hudson Street, New York, NY 10014.

a member of
Penguin Group (USA) Inc.
375 Hudson Street
New York, NY 10014
www.penguin.com

Library of Congress Cataloging-in-Publication Data

Fromm, Mallory, date.
Qi energy for health and healing : a comprehensive guide to accessing
your healing energy / Mallory Fromm.
p. cm.
Includes index.
ISBN 1-58333-157-3
1. Qi gong. 2. Qi gong—Health aspects. 3. Physical fitness. I. Title.
RA781.8.F763   2003   2002043998
613.7'1—dc21

Printed in the United States of America
1 3 5 7 9 10 8 6 4 2

BOOK DESIGN BY DEBORAH KERNER/DANCING BEARS DESIGN

Energy is Eternal Delight
Exuberance is Beauty

WILLIAM BLAKE

TO THERESE AND CORIN
Who embody the Beauty of Exuberance

ACKNOWLEDGMENTS

Pamela Hartman was the ideal illustrator. As well as being a skilled artist, she is an accomplished bodywork professional certified in the Alexander Technique and physio-synthesis. Her knowledge of holistic medicine and human anatomy made our collaboration easy and fruitful. She managed to care for an ailing mother, a nagging author, and needy patients with impeccable aplomb, and still meet her deadline. I am grateful to her.

For twenty-five years, Hidehiko Suzuki, the most humane man I have ever met, has enriched my life with his humor, intellect, and compassion. His infectious optimism and encouragement saw me through many not-so-quiet moments of desperation during the writing of this book. I hope that my enduring gratitude is worthy of his enduring friendship.

LOS ANGELES
August 2002

Contents

Foreword   *xiii*
Introduction   *1*

PART I   **What Is Qi?**

CHAPTER 1.   ALL ABOUT QI   *11*
Healthy Energy   *11*
Traditional Eastern Medicine   *13*
Introducing Qi   *14*
Obsessed with Illness   *16*
Qi and Health   *18*

CHAPTER 2.   ACCESSING AND APPLYING YOUR QI   *22*
Warming Up   *22*
Basic Procedure   *24*
Intermediate Procedure   *28*
Advanced Procedure   *31*
Paired Technique   *32*
Concentrating and Transmitting Your Qi   *33*
Relaxing the Mind/Body Unity   *38*
Qi for Pets   *41*
Applying Your Qi   *44*
The Most Common Question   *50*

CHAPTER 3.   OUR LATENT POWER   *52*

Adapting and Adjusting   *52*

How the Body Adapts   *53*

Stress and the Flow of Qi   *58*

A Question of Balance   *59*

The Extrapyramidal Motor System and

the Autonomic Nervous System   *60*

I Encounter *Kiryū*   *63*

You Encounter *Kiryū*   *66*

Solitary *Kiryū*   *68*

Tales of *Kiryū*   *73*

PART II   **Using the Healing Power of Qi**

CHAPTER 4.   THE SPINE AND BODY SYSTEMS   *77*

Digestion   *77*

Body Cleansing   *85*

Muscles and Bones   *97*

Seasonal Change and Fine-Tuning   *108*

Biorhythms   *113*

Sleep   *116*

CHAPTER 5.   PREGNANCY AND CHILDBIRTH   *126*

Qi for Two   *126*

Thoughts on Pregnancy   *127*

The Baby Palace   *128*

Qi and the Pregnant Woman   *130*

The First Trimester   *132*

The Second Trimester   *145*

The Third Trimester   *159*

Childbirth   *162*

After Giving Birth   *164*

CHAPTER 6. THE VERY YOUNG AND THE VERY OLD   *167*
The First Years   *167*
Newborns   *169*
Infants, Toddlers, and Young Children   *172*
The Elderly   *177*

CHAPTER 7. SEXUALITY   *186*
Sexual Energy   *186*
Qi Treatment for Premature Aging
   and for Restoring Sexual Energy   *191*

CHAPTER 8. QI AND THE ULTIMATE TRANSITION   *196*
A Parable   *196*
Caretaking of the Terminally Ill and Elderly   *197*
Final Guidance   *202*
Sublimed Qi   *205*
How I Would Like to Die   *208*
How I Try to Live   *211*

Appendix A: A Handy Guide to the Spine   *212*
Appendix B: A Handy Guide to the Head   *215*
Index   *217*

FOREWORD

I completed my college education in France and took a higher degree in England. When I began my twenty-year career of living, working, and studying in Japan, I often wondered why my fate landed me in the opposite direction from where my youthful ambitions had led me. I had a "significant other" living there whom I eventually married, and so you might say that my heart led me to Japan. However, early on I wondered what my soul would find there.

The answer is, of course, qi. For brevity's sake, I will not go into the numerous applications and implications of qi that I use in daily life and in my practice as a holistic health-care practitioner. Letting qi guide me through a perfect late-in-life pregnancy changed my perspective and approach to health.

I had already been an avid believer in the power of qi and an enthusiastic fan of the wonderful practitioners I encountered in Japan, beginning with the redoubtable Kayoko Matsuura. During the process of pregnancy and birth, I exercised my qi more than ever before, and I was rewarded not only with a beautiful child, but also with a new faith in my own strength. I now exercise my qi when I work, when I garden, when I care for my elderly mother. I even use it to help me choose clothing or a new car. Not that everyone will care to exercise her qi for grocery shopping, but the innate and latent power is there.

Carl Jung had a Latin quote inscribed over the door to his Zurich home: *Vocatus atque non vocatus Deus aderit* (Bidden or unbidden, God is there). I would substitute *Qi* for the word *Deus:* Bidden or unbidden, Qi is there. Your own quiet, powerful tool to help guide you through a healthy life, and beyond, lies literally at your fingertips.

In this book, my husband, Dr. Mallory Fromm, has given the Western reader a concise, systematic, and practical tool to the understanding and treatment of pain management, preventive health care, and health maintenance by using qi. I believe it is a supremely useful resource for reassuring the average person that she can take charge of her own health. Many practitioners in Japan consider this discipline to be their finest cultural export, surpassing woodblock prints, Noh, Kabuki, and sumo. So do I.

To me this book represents an elegant expression of our lives and studies during more than twenty years in Japan. My heart is completely satisfied in a marriage to a loving teacher and gifted writer. My soul is gratified in my knowledge of health and healing, and in my ability to pass that knowledge on to others.

THERESE BAXTER
Tokyo
March 2002

Qi Energy
for Health and Healing

Introduction

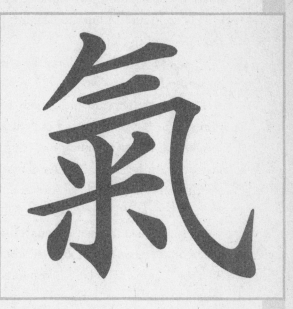

I Encounter Qi

My first encounter with qi occurred when I was an undergraduate student at London University, learning things Japanese and Chinese. The encounter was neither memorable nor particularly influential in my life. Qi (pronounced *chi* in Chinese, and *ki* in Japanese and Korean) was one more Chinese character (*kanji*) to learn; one of about 3,000 that I was forced to fix indelibly in my brain.

It happened to be one of the most popular *kanji* in the vocabulary, and I remember thinking as a freshman how versatile qi was. It was used in *kanji* compounds for *health, illness, electricity, sanity, madness, strength/weakness of character, weather, purpose, energy, feelings, courage,* and a myriad more. It was hard to make a simple declarative sentence without fitting qi in, and it was impossible to discuss anything physical or emotional without resorting to qi several times. The ubiquity of qi within the language and culture struck me as interesting, but no more than that.

The construction of the *kanji* is divided into two parts, the outer part and the inner part. The former signifies vapor, steam, gas . . . invisible yet potent energy. The latter is the *kanji* for "rice," the staple food of Asia. "Okay, so we eat food (fuel), which produces invisible energy, and that is how we exist," I thought, unimpressed, and then passed on to the next *kanji* to be learned. If I subsequently thought about the *kanji* for qi at all, the fatal result of the absence of fuel seemed so obvious and inevitable that I did not consider its philosophical implications. "No rice/fuel equals starvation" was all that occurred to me.

Today, I think that life is the presence of qi, and death is the absence of qi. I have no better definition.

While still a student, I briefly took up the martial art Aikido, which I had heard rumored to be based on the mental and physical properties of qi. The word *Aikido* means "the way of blending qis," but my qi did not at all blend with that of my first instructor. In Japanese, the blending of qis means to get along well with someone, and our qis could not have been further apart. I gave up on him, but not on Aikido.

Coming to Japan as a research student pursuing a doctorate at London University, I had another encounter with qi. This encounter was indeed memorable.

I once again attempted Aikido training, and this time I stayed. My instructor, Takeshi Watabe, who later became recognized as a master of the discipline, and who taught and practiced with vigor into his late eighties, had qi with which mine blended seamlessly. I spent twenty-seven happy years under his tutelage. It was he who defined the essence of Aikido as "the right move at the right time." It might well be the recipe for a happy life. Certainly, recognizing the link between qi and timing (in its widest and deepest implications) gave my mind and body something to chew on.

My third encounter with qi occurred as I was just on the verge of completing my doctoral thesis. This encounter resulted in an ongoing love affair with qi that influenced the course of my life.

As I was putting the final high gloss on my dissertation, I suffered a physical breakdown. Perhaps *letdown* would be a better word. I had never given my body a second thought, but had taken its health and vitality for granted, and so the fact that it "gave out on me," reducing me to intense pain and a bedridden condition, seemed like an inexplicable betrayal.

The decline in my physical condition went hand in hand with a drop in my spirits. My outlook plummeted. To say that I was pessimistic and depressed would be an understatement. My only really active mood was desperation. I sometimes had dreams in which I made a Faustian pact with some devil whereby I would commit a horrible crime in return for being released from pain and regaining mobility.

A detailed account of my illness, cure, and awakening to the health-giving virtues of qi has been published elsewhere. Here, I will only summarize by saying that, after two fruitless and frustrating years of trying a dozen physicians and a dozen holistic (alternative) practitioners, including acupuncturists and chiropractors, I was finally healed by an eighty-year-old Japanese woman in about thirty minutes. She diagnosed my problem using qi and healed my ailment using qi. I became her ardent admirer and pupil.

Her name was Kayoko Matsuura, and she was one practitioner among many—certainly the most gifted—of a Japanese holistic health organization that employs a modern revision of classical Chinese healing and health techniques based on qi. She introduced me to the world of healing qi, which, when appended to the martial qi I had been studying, created a vital totality of "the right move at the right time." She used to kid me that I could beat someone to a pulp, and then heal him, something along the lines of the legendary Japanese man of medicine known as Red Beard.

Mrs. Matsuura practiced her art without letup until she died at the age of eighty-five. Though she had experienced what the Japanese call a "sublime death," I was, of course, saddened, and when my sadness passed, it was time to find a new teacher after having learned from her for four years.

I took courses at the health organization and joined small "study groups" of other practitioner-hopefuls. Eventually, I was able to learn directly from a practitioner whom Mrs. Matsuura had always spoken of with the highest regard. It was never my goal to practice any healing or health maintenance; quite the opposite. I continued my study of qi out of intellectual curiosity and interest, because it gave me a sense of health and well-being, and in order to attend to the health needs of my immediate family. Beyond that, I had no ambition. I was living half the year in Japan, and so could just learn and practice for my own sake.

It happened that, about nine years into my study, a sixty-year-old Japanese friend came to see me socially and complained of chronic shoulder pain. He had been diagnosed as having an advanced case of bursitis, was told his condition was hopeless, and that he should consider having surgery. I impulsively asked him to let me have a go at alleviating his pain, he agreed, and his shoulder condition cleared up in two days. On the fourth day following his visit, my phone began ringing and people began turning up at my door asking to be treated. After I got over my surprise, my reactions were mixed. Half of me was flustered and lacked confidence; the other half was gratified and eager to get to work. Through an unforeseen event, I had a practice in spite of myself.

The practice has been thriving since that day both in the United States and in Japan.

You Encounter Qi

I would like you to encounter qi through my experience.

I was diagnosed as having a herniated disc between my third and fourth lumbar vertebrae, which caused me exquisite nerve pain called sciatica. Of the dozen physicians I approached, not one of them gave me a different diagnosis, nor did one of them say anything other than my body was in terrible shape. At least half expressed grave concern for me, and a couple of orthopedic surgeons suggested an immediate surgical procedure, called a laminectomy, to fuse my vertebrae.

Kayoko Matsuura had me lie supine on the floor. She looked at me carefully, had me turn over, and placed her hand over the spot of the herniated disc.

She said, "You've got a very good body. It has great resilience, and is always working hard to stay healthy."

"Well, it sure failed with my lower back," I said ruefully.

"There is nothing the matter with your lower back," she replied, casually flicking away two years of my life like a piece of lint. "You have a problem with your ankle."

She proceeded to heal me, and as she did so, she baffled me with her "logic." She told me that my outer left ankle had risen about an inch, exposing a cluster of nerves. My body, in order to avoid great pain, changed its center of gravity, which led to a change of posture, thus causing me to walk differently. At the same time, this change in posture and gait signaled my third lumbar vertebra to twist and press against the sciatic nerve, creating my pain. The vertebra did this in order to "help" me, since the sciatic pain was less than what the ankle, foot, and shin pain would have been. In other words, one part of me came to the aid of another part of me in order to do good by stealth. I was completely unaware of this good deed.

That "explanation" sounded nutty to me, and I am sure it sounds nutty to you.

However, her treatment worked. When she lowered the ankle, the third lumbar vertebra untwisted naturally, and the sciatic pain went away.

"You mean two dozen people looked no further than your spine?" Kayoko Matsuura asked in astonishment. "Without fixing your ankle, nothing could help your back or leg."

"I was close to getting a laminectomy," I said thoughtfully, half to myself, and looked at her gratefully.

She smiled, and her lined face creased up like an old paper bag. To me, she looked gorgeous.

"Welcome to the life of qi," she said, and left me to work on the next person.

The fact that my spine responded in a "helpful way" to my ankle's predicament was the reason she told me I had a resilient, health-seeking body. She called that response a positive adaptation to a certain stimulus. She diagnosed the origin of my sciatica using qi, and produced a healing response by the application of qi. She also told me that my original "helpful" response was produced by the beneficial workings of qi; that she had used her qi on mine to produce a positive adaptation that led me to heal.

I remained baffled by her logic until I learned more about qi. I was not alone. Few of those whom she healed could make heads or tails of her "logic." I propose to take you, the reader, from that initial stage of universal bafflement to a broad understanding of just what that remarkable woman was talking about.

There is no single, definitive definition of health and well-being. No matter how "objectively and absolutely" your health is measured, it is always qualified "subjectively and relatively." Your blood can be drawn and your various values printed out, but then you are evaluated by age, sex, other psycho/physical variables, and finally, how you look and feel. Depending on what you eat, drink, and dream (i.e., sleep well or poorly), the values can change radically in a week. The abundance or dearth of stress in your life will also cause a considerable change in the values of your blood. Simply receiving unexpected good news will make you seem, from the inside, like a different person.

I believe that health and well-being are a matter of how much satisfaction you take in life. I do not mean by this simply freedom from pain or discomfort. I am talking about a more positive, more vigorous sense of being alive. One's quality of life; the pleasure obtained just by being alive; the curiosity, interest, and appreciation one brings to living . . . these are what health and well-being consist of, with or without pain.

Our quality of life is, physiologically, based on our bodies' reactions and responses to external stimuli. Not only are our five senses constantly barraged by stimuli, but so are our immune system, gastrointestinal system, pulmonary system, cardiovascular system, and so on. A stressful business meeting can cause a harmful elevation of blood pressure. At the same time, it can cause the stomach to secrete excessive acid. The entire body, beginning with the cardiovascular and digestive systems, must react and respond to this physiological fact.

On the other hand, the sweet scent of a blooming rose or the sight of a spectacular sunset can cause a healthy drop in our blood pressure and our digestive organs to purr.

A healthy body is one that responds appropriately to the myriad stimuli it encounters. It must *adapt* to an unending series of changes ("the right move at the right time"). On a large, almost glacially slow scale, our bodies adapt to changes in season. We go into a summer mode, which is different from a winter mode. The body expands and loosens in the summer, and contracts and tightens in the winter. On a tiny, extremely fast scale, we inhale an irritating fragment, say a grain of pepper, and we sneeze it out. This, too, is a healthy adaptation to a change in circumstances. Were it not for that sneeze, the nasal passages would become inflamed.

Thus, the finer the power of adaptation, the healthier we are and the more we enjoy life.

One of the goals of this book is to enlighten readers to their own *adaptive power*. By becoming aware of the circumstances and ways in which our bodies adapt to different stimuli, we also become aware of just how sensitive our bodies are, how eager they are to do us good service (if only we let them), and how much latent power is lying dormant in us waiting to be roused into action on behalf of our health and well-being.

In short, I seek to acquaint the reader with his or her own qi. It is through accessing, manipulating, and observing the working of qi, both in ourselves and in others, that we refine our adaptive power and realize our latent power. If "knowledge is power," then "knowledge of power" is knowledge devoutly to be wished. For *power,* read *qi.*

It is on this point, I believe, that my outlook differs from that of most "alternative" or "holistic" practitioners. They seek to impose health on the body from without by administering regular treatment, food and mineral supplements, or a "healthy regimen" that usually binds the patient to them. I seek to call forth the latent power from within so that the individual is eventually freed from reliance on external sources. The individual becomes, as he or she was intended to be, self-sufficient in health.

It is my conviction based on years of experience and observation that the power for good and enduring health is latent in all of us. As I stated earlier, life is the presence of qi. This being so, it requires only an awareness, strengthening, and refining of our qi to bring out the healthiest in us. I say *only* as a form of encouragement, because being healthy is not at all tedious. Quite the opposite. How to engage your qi and the qi of others and the health benefits that accrue from that engagement will be enlarged upon during the course of the book.

It is my intention to provide a wide-ranging view of human health and behavior according to the workings of qi. I seek ultimately to free the individual from total reliance on external health care by placing the facility to "help thyself" literally at the reader's fingertips. This book is designed to be informative and practical, and so contains only an occasional nugget of philosophy. These nuggets may be ignored or stored away like a squirrel's winter nuts to be savored at a later date.

The only topics I have chosen not to address are those that allopathic medicine deals with so very well: surgery, emergency, and pharmaceuticals. This book in no way sets itself up in opposition to Western medicine, either in principle or in practice. The cowman and the sheepman could be friends, and so can the physician and the holistic practitioner. Nor will I describe the body in terms of longitudes, latitudes, meridians, chakras, and other non-Western terms. The simple biology and physiology presented here are the very same you learned in high school, if not earlier.

This book is designed to be read, experienced, and enjoyed by the intelligent amateur. The treatments presented are not as complex or elaborate as one would encounter at a professional qi treatment. On the other hand, they are more than superficial. They require concentration and patience, not to mention more than a little goodwill. I have erred on the side of conservatism in the time I allocate for each treatment and procedure. The more skillful one becomes with qi, the faster the treatments progress and the stronger the responses become.

Each treatment presented in this book is meant to be performed in a single session and in the order of appearance of the body parts to be treated. I have organized the treatments to make them as effective as possible. Regular repetition of treatment, say two or three times a week over the course of a month, will promote the lasting benefits of the treatment.

I hope, by the end of the book, to have provided a comprehensive, elegant, logical, and practical view of the human body—its creation, growth, maturity, decline, and demise—through the eyes of our natural energy.

PART I

What Is
Qi?

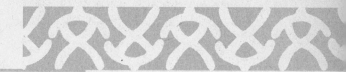

CHAPTER 1

All About Qi

Healthy Energy

By healthy energy I mean positive feelings that fill one with optimism and warmth, even enthusiasm. It is the excitement and buoyancy you feel when you receive unexpected good news. That excitement and buoyancy quickly communicate themselves to others, who can become as giddy and happy as you are.

Healthy energy is, therefore, infectious and contagious. I use the words ironically, because they are usually associated with disease and illness.

I am sure you have at one time or another experienced the following. You are at a party or gathering where the atmosphere is pleasant, congenial, and charged with energy. One or two people enter the room, speak to one or two other guests who then speak to other guests, and within minutes, the atmosphere has changed dramatically. It is as if all the energy has been sucked out of the room, and you wonder how you had been enjoying yourself earlier. The room has become "infected" with low energy. The people whose presence transformed the party are themselves transformed. They appear to be gaining energy as you and your fellow guests lose yours.

This is a classic example of negative or unhealthy energy. People possessed of negative energy feed upon the healthy energy of others in order to exist. It is a form of vampirism. In fact, such people do not so much infect you with unhealthy energy as deplete you of healthy energy.

On the other hand, everyone knows a person who "lights up a room" with his or her presence. Someone who has a "magnetic personality." Someone who makes you feel good just by standing near you. Someone who gives you a feeling of well-being with a smile.

This is a classic example of infectious or contagious healthy energy. A meeting of healthy energies leaves both parties feeling physically, mentally, and emotionally stimulated in a very pleasant way.

Destiny may determine whom you meet, but it is the convergence of healthy energies that determines with whom you fall in love. Marriage may be made for any number of logical, rational, and self-serving reasons. But love, as our poets, novelists, artists, and composers have told us through the ages, refuses to fit into a logical pigeonhole. It is the great inexplicable act of our lives.

Once again, let us call the act of falling in love the convergence of healthy energies. Or to put it another way, the happiest working of qi. Healthy energy or potent qi is like love, in that it is not self-seeking, but other-seeking. It also possesses the Byronic quality of love as "an enlargement of existence." Our very existence and our awareness of it enlarge and deepen with the healthy, energetic state of love.

Qi is our natural energy, our healthy energy. Obviously, we are not going to fall in love on a regular basis, but we can go through life with the awareness that a healthy energy is one that is not self-seeking, but is, rather, selfless and inclined to generosity toward others. A mother will put her life at risk to save her child, despite the fact that it would be more prudent and rational to walk the other way.

I am not advising anyone to consciously adopt a self-sacrificing outlook. It comes naturally when we care for someone or something. We willingly and gladly subsume our self within the larger entity of love, and put that love foremost. People who love their country willingly die for it. The same holds true for a love of truth or a love of God. Romeo and Juliet cannot live without each other. I believe that an intention to do good or to help another results in a strong, effective flow of qi both within you and in the transmission of your healthy energy.

Traditional Eastern Medicine

Using qi for medical purposes has been pursued in Asia since ancient times, and has been systematized into several major forms of treatment. In particular, patterns of breathing and breath control were seen early on to determine the flow or blockage of qi. Indeed, esteeming breath as synonymous with qi and its purity is still fundamental to, and vital in, yoga and qi gong as well as other disciplines of the Asian healing canon.

More and more Westerners are finding alternative forms of health and medicine to their liking. In the United States, more consumers pay out of pocket for alternative medicine than for allopathic. The trend is growing strong enough to warrant coverage by insurance companies in some cases.

Most Westerners, however, still take the "If it ain't broke why fix it?" approach to their bodies, and so come into contact with "medical" qi more for healing than for preventive medicine and health maintenance. For example, acupuncture is based on the flow of qi along "meridians" that run through the body, and has been found to produce relief from various aches and pains. The same is true for acupressure and shiatsu. As a result, all three enjoy widespread popularity as *remedies*.

This use of medicine on a "Now it's broke, let's fix it" basis unfortunately falls far short of the Eastern model of prevention and health maintenance. The average American is zealous in upholding the Eastern paradigm where his automobile is concerned. People change oil, get new tires, get tune-ups, lube jobs, fresh water and fluids, and regularly have their brakes checked for wear and tear though there is not the slightest indication of an irregularity.

What I am introducing in this book is the concept of treating yourself and your family even better than you treat your car. I am seeking to convince you to adopt an alternative method of achieving, improving, and maintaining health.

As stated in the Introduction, the *kanji* for qi is made of two parts. The outer part symbolizes a vapor, such as steam, representing energy. The inner part is rice. Life is created and sustained through the fuel (rice) being transformed into energy (steam). In the Asian healing tradition, this process is represented by the cycle of breath.

Look at the humanesque or lionesque or grotesque guardian figures in front of Chinese and Japanese temples. There are always two, one with mouth open, one with mouth closed. One is inhaling and the other is exhaling. They represent the continuous cycle of life-sustaining breath, made audible by the sounds *ah* (inhale) and *un* (exhale).

The pursuit and systematization of qi has not been undertaken in the West, which is not to say that there is no tradition of qi in the West. According to Genesis, God breathed life into Adam. This breathing is significant since breath, potent but invisible, is a metaphor for qi as well as the physical means of accessing and transmitting qi. The instrument of transmission is the finger or fingerlike object.

The qi/breath of God and its transmission are wonderfully illustrated by Michelangelo's fresco of the act of creation, painted on the ceiling of the Sistine Chapel in the Vatican. The powerful arm of the Creator is thrust out to instill breath into the lifeless body of Adam. See how the muscular, confident hand of God contrasts with Adam's limp, dangling wrist. You can practically feel the qi/breath passing between the finger of Life-That-Is and the finger of Life-to-Be.

"And the Lord God formed man of the dust of the ground, and breathed into his nostrils the breath of life; and man became a living soul."

The concept and power of qi have never had a better nor more eloquent testimonial.

What I have just written is meant to reassure the reader that though qi medicine is an import from the East, it is neither exotic nor alien. It can become a part of your life as easily as sushi, tai chi, and quality circles have become in the lives of many Westerners.

Introducing Qi

Having, I hope, put a homespun, friendly face on qi, it is time to describe it and explain its workings.

The term *qi energy* is a redundancy like *rich billionaire.* Qi is energy in any and all of its guises and forms. It is the electricity that lights up a room or emblazons the sky. It is the electromagnetism that envelops Earth. It is the crisp vitality you feel after a good night's sleep on the first day of your vacation. It regulates the unconscious activity of internal and external organs that you never notice until the activity is somehow impeded. It is manifested in the love you feel for the kind and caring, and the hatred you feel for the wicked and cruel. Desire, loathing, pity, envy, joy . . . all are expressions of qi.

We are imbued with qi from the moment of conception, in fact, prior to conception thanks to our components of creation: the living sperm wriggles into the waiting egg by the energy of qi. We retain qi until the moment of death. And unlike our muscles and organs, the quality of our qi is not inevitably bound to deteriorate or erode with age. Our qi does not peter out as our hearing and vision fail. In fact, it is interesting to note that contrary to "logic," qi does not ebb out of us during our progress toward death, nor vanish at the moment of death. It seeks to reassert itself during our final waning of life, and so bursts out from us at intervals. This accounts for the sudden manic deathbed behavior of people who rewrite wills and harass their poor relations. Our literature is full of such suddenly rejuvenated characters.

What is more common is the inexplicable (albeit temporary) "remissions" or bursts of energy when all hope has passed. This is the activity of qi as the organism gravitates toward death. At the moment of death, there is an efflorescence of qi, not unlike the last flaring of a guttering candle. Then, poof . . .

Pathological examination of living tissue and recently deceased tissue will find no observable differences. Yet one specimen will be from a living person and the other from a corpse. The difference is the presence or absence of qi; the former still has qi, while the latter no longer does. This is what makes organ transplants possible: the qi has departed and the organism is pronounced "dead," but the tissue goes on living. That living tissue can then be maintained by the qi of someone else.

Qi is, therefore, the essence of life, which is why it is frequently (and clumsily) called *life force* or *vital energy.* Stated less dramatically, qi is what informs the existence of every living thing. (Earlier, I rendered qi as natural energy and healthy energy in English. Those terms seem less daunting than *life force* and *vital energy.* Qi is as easy to get to know and like as ice cream, and far less fattening.)

It is easy to mistake the raw substance for the spirit that animates it. Our bodies (the biblical "dust") are brought to life and kept alive through the energy of qi until the moment qi is terminated. And, if you believe in the physics principle of the conservation of energy, our qi is not terminated by death, but is transmuted into some other form of energy within the cosmos. Who knows but that there may even be a pool of qi in the universe from which we come and to which we return. Certainly, Hindu philosophy and the concept of rebirth would not find this idea alien or outlandish.

This being the case, to return to the theme of love, "we were made for each other" might actually be "we were made from each other."

I fear I have strayed from my subject. It is obvious that qi is *universal* in that each and every living one of us has it, as do our pets and plants. Qi is *specific* insofar as we each have a certain body type and character that both modifies and is modified by qi. We all sleep, eat, and excrete, but it is doubtful that you know anyone whose eating, sleeping, and toileting behaviors are exactly like yours.

In the same way, people complain of being unable to find "like-minded" people. In the culture of the East, people whose qis "blend" are like-minded and become friends for life, while those whose qis fail to blend should not take the trouble to try and get to know each other. The effort is doomed to failure.

Obsessed with Illness

There were lymph glands that might do him in. There were kidneys, nerve sheaths and corpuscles. There were tumors of the brain. There was Hodgkin's disease, leukemia, amyotrophic lateral sclerosis. There were fertile red meadows of epithelial tissue to catch and coddle a cancer cell. There were diseases of the skin, diseases of the bone, diseases of the lung, diseases of the stomach, diseases of the heart, blood and arteries. There were diseases of the head, diseases of the neck, diseases of the chest, diseases of the intestines, diseases of the crotch. There were even diseases of the feet. There were billions of conscientious body cells oxidating away day and night like dumb animals at their complicated job of keeping him alive and healthy, and every one was a potential traitor and foe.

He wondered often how he would ever recognize the first chill, flush, twinge, ache, belch, sneeze, stain, lethargy, vocal slip, loss of balance or lapse of memory that would signal the inevitable beginning of the inevitable end.

—JOSEPH HELLER, *Catch-22*

Western medicine treats illness, not health. No one but a lunatic would visit the doctor to boast of feeling terrific. Physicians can say in all honesty that they wish they could eradicate every disease just as polio and smallpox were eradicated. However, that would put roughly a half million physicians out of work overnight in America alone. Think of ancillary health-care providers and all the foundations, corporations, pharmaceutical companies, publishing companies, and medical schools whose existence is premised on the inevitability of disease, illness, and debility through aging, and you can readily understand why illness, rather than the prevention of illness, is a national obsession.

The human body is viewed as an illness waiting to happen, and people rush to have tests taken at the first twinge or second sneeze. Of course, the potential for a debilitating or fatal illness is always present, but likewise, a fatal crash is always potential in a car or airplane trip for as many factors as contribute to succumbing to an illness.

With so much money and energy and media coverage invested in illness, it is easy to overlook a very simple fact: the human body always strives toward health. This striving for health may not always be successful; for many reasons, the individual physiology frequently falls short of success. That does not mean, however, that the body does not actively do its utmost to help itself. In twenty years of studying and practicing Far Eastern medicine, I have never encountered a body that sought to self-destruct, nor have I ever encountered a body that did not gravitate to health over illness.

Let us take a simple and quite common occurrence: A fertile woman has a breast lumpectomy, the tissue is found to be malignant, the woman undergoes chemotherapy, and is subsequently pronounced "clean." She then has to wait out a five-year survival period, during which time she dreads the recurrence of the cancer.

Let us look at the same phenomenon in another way. First, the woman's physiological equilibrium was thrown off balance by cancer. Her body then received two blows: the first was psychological (being notified of the existence of a potentially fatal cancer); the second was physical (undergoing an invasive surgical procedure that left a scar). Following this, the body was flooded with chemicals so powerful that hair falls out and natural body cleansing (menstruation) is impeded. Finally, the woman is filled with dread and anxiety, which are manifested in poor sleeping and digestion, a loss of energy, and a decline in her enjoyment of daily life.

Her body has its work cut out for it. It seeks the restoration of health by working from the most recent problem backward to the original problem. It is like peeling off a layer to reveal another layer to reveal another layer until the body returns to the cancerous lump in the breast. Now with the lump absent, the body can turn its attention elsewhere.

In other words, the woman's body will (1) seek a release from anxiety and dread in order to sleep and digest better, (2) seek to reenergize its natural cleansing system through menstruation and such detoxification functions as sweating and excreting in order to purge itself of any residual chemicals, (3) seek to repair tissue damage caused by surgery, (4) seek to release the original shock/blow she received upon hearing the diagnosis of cancer, and (5) seek to defend itself from future cancer by means of its immune system.

Qi treatment will vastly speed up this recovery process by channeling and intensifying the woman's natural and latent healing energies. Her body can be specifically directed and induced to heal itself to the best of its ability.

Qi and Health

Considering the specificity of qi leads us to the topic of health. A physical or objective standard of health—in other words, what is healthy and what is not—is at best a statistic and at worst an illusion.

It is possible to list factors promoting longevity, but is longevity synonymous with health? My grandfather lived almost to ninety, but his life, prolonged by what the physician called "heroic measures," had nothing healthy about it. It is not stated how Methuselah felt when he turned nine hundred, but one has only to look at the majority of the modern elderly to see that survival has little to do with health.

Nor do bulging biceps and taut thighs, much less buns of steel: the so-called hardbodies. It is a sign of just how far our civilization has lost sight of health that impressive appearance is valued above holistic integrity. People today have confused fitness with health, and so strive to mold their bodies into objects suited to being sold in hardware stores. It is an aesthetic goal, not a health program.

You may be able to run ten kilometers wearing a twenty-five-pound backpack, but the contingency of your having to do this in daily life is remote. Health is what it takes to deal and cope comfortably with the exigencies, traumas, dramas, and joys of daily life. Fitness, other than for those who are paid to be fit—professional athletes, policemen, firemen, soldiers, and so on—is vanity. Not that vanity is bad. Not at all. For some, it is all they have to live for. But it should be recognized as vanity, and should not be confused with a mission of health. Flabby men and scrawny women may have wonderful health, while fitness enthusiasts may suffer all sorts of aches and pains, or worse, have little or no physical sensitivity.

The keys to health are flexibility and resilience, which lifting, tensing, and repetitive movements do nothing to promote. There is a Confucian saying: *The Superior Person is not a utensil,* meaning capable of one use only. It is of greater benefit to health to have a lively immune system, a reliable metabolism, and the ability to recover quickly from blows, both physical and emotional, than muscles capable of bench-pressing four hundred pounds.

Let us concede that there is no paradigm of health, and let us also concede that it is just as likely a healthy person would get that way without any particular "health regimen" as with one. Genes, DNA, anatomy . . . physiological factors that function as what used to be called "destiny" are more likely to promote or impede health than megadoses of vitamins.

What, then, is a useful definition of health, and how does it relate to the activity of qi? *Health is the satisfaction one takes in life.* People are awarded prizes on television for longevity, for living to be a hundred years old and more, as if they had masterminded and executed a plan to reach that great age. No prizes go to people who, through a fortuitous chemistry of genes, character, and environment, lead a wholly satisfying life no matter how short.

Life is unfair. Some are born with bodies that can swill gin and chain-smoke cigarettes and live happily to a hundred, while others are born to a physiology that can digest nothing stronger than crackers and milk, and who eke out a short life. This anatomical inequality may strike some people as un-American; they would like the "all men are created equal" concept to apply to the organism as well as to the citizen. Yet this organic inequality is paraded before us daily: the tall, the short, the handsome, the ugly, the intelligent, the dim-witted, and so on.

More subtle are the "gifts" some people have. People may have a gift for math, or for music, or for learning foreign languages, or for drawing. Some people have gifted constitutions.

We all have physiological limitations—our anatomical destinies—and while health programs and regimens may supplement those limitations, they cannot alter them. The pills, diets, lifestyles, accessories, and treatments that are sold to us either state outright or imply that they can overcome our innate limitations. Alas, they cannot.

These innate limitations frustrate us terribly. We complain that we are not as healthy as we used to be. However, it is the aging process that brings our limitations into clear definition. We might as well complain that we do not grow younger with age. We forget that there is such a thing as healthy aging, which takes the current condition of the mind/body into account after (in the words of statisticians) adjusting for age.

I meet people suffering from all sorts of afflictions—stroke, heart attack, cancer, sciatica, scoliosis—who tell me they are not healthy. Yet many of these people nevertheless take immense satisfaction in life, in the activity of being alive. *Health is the flexibility and resilience to deal with what physically and emotionally befalls us,* whether it be an unforeseen car accident, an illness, or the death of a loved one. As in the case of the elderly, these people are as healthy as they can be given their circumstances.

What qi treatment does is to bring the body to its full potential for health. If you have a lemon body, so be it. Nothing can alter that. However, qi treatment can give you the best lemon body you can possibly attain. Those crackers and milk will taste better after treatment, and become surprisingly nutritious. And if you are blessed with a sound mind and body, qi treatment provides regular tune-ups to keep you at the top of your physical and mental form.

In other words, the correct application of qi allows you to fulfill your physiological potential. Thus, the ultimate goal of qi treatment is not longevity or muscular development or an improved IQ, but the attainment of a physical/mental state in which it is possible to have a vigorous appreciation of life. In the world of health according to qi, quality, not quantity, is the way to go.

Qi is a wonderful means of alleviating or eliminating aches and pains, as well as healing a wide range of ailments and afflictions. Moreover, after qi treatment, many people, myself included, report a sensation of euphoria or happiness or just plain exuberance. It's the invigorating, life-affirming feeling of receiving unexpected good news, the good news being that your body has reached its current potential for health and feels great. The sensation lifts you out of whatever rut you had landed and were stranded in.

Half the people I treat walk in saying that they feel great and want to maintain that feeling. Healing illnesses and making people feel better not withstanding, maintaining their awareness of health is what is most gratifying about my practice.

CHAPTER 2

Accessing and Applying Your Qi

Warming Up

As in the case of learning any new skill or technique, accessing your qi may seem at first mannered and even labored. However, with daily practice, you will be able to access and concentrate your qi quickly and effortlessly within a week to ten days. At that point, the procedure that follows may be modified or abandoned, and you may want to proceed to the intermediate and advanced techniques for accessing your qi.

You will be using touch and breath to access your qi. It is, therefore, necessary to be in the proper environment. That means a calm, quiet space where you feel comfortable and are able to relax. You may want to play some soothing or familiar music in order to clear your mind of extraneous thoughts.

"When the mind's free, the body's delicate," said Shakespeare, and I couldn't have put it better myself.

The key to the successful and effective access of qi is mind/body relaxation.

Once you achieve familiarity with accessing your qi, you will have powers of concentration that will allow you to access it in almost any environment and under almost any circumstances. (I've done it underwater, but hesitate to try it while riding a roller coaster.) Since accessing your qi is a simple and effective means to mind/body relaxation, it is always good to try to find a space congenial to that end, with or without music.

Sit comfortably with both feet planted squarely and firmly on the floor. Let gravity support your lower body and spine. Sit as erect as possible without feeling any discomfort. You are not expected to assume a military posture, but a slumping posture will be a hindrance to concentration. It is preferable, but not absolutely necessary, to sit without leaning your back against anything. This posture provides an awareness of the amount of tension or relaxation in your upper body and spine.

For those seeking an authentic Far Eastern experience regardless of discomfort and pain, you may sit on the floor (bare boards or concrete flooring for extreme thrillseekers) on your knees with your backside resting on your heels. Within a minute you will feel a tingling in your lower body, which should not be confused with the feeling of accessing qi. You are experiencing the telltale signs of an interrupted blood supply. Fiery pain will soon follow. Some people claim that speed of access is greatly enhanced through this posture, as they race to concentrate their qi before the torment begins. I myself prefer to stand or sit comfortably and let the relaxation that accrues from this exercise linger.

Let us assume, then, that you are sitting erect with your spine supported from its base rather than by the back of a chair. Both feet are flat on the floor. Be aware of how your head is resting on the neck. It should be straight, supported by the spine, and not leaning to one side or another. Your face should be pointing straight ahead. It is time to feel for tension in your neck and shoulders. There is bound to be some. Take a deep breath and exhale slowly, letting your shoulders sink. At the same time, let your hands find a natural and comfortable position on your lap (see Figure 2.1).

Breathe naturally and easily for half a minute. Be aware of your breathing and whether you feel any tension in your chest, especially around your solar plexus (between the two sides of the rib cage and beneath the breastbone). Should you feel tension, deepen your breathing and prolong your exhalations. Stress induces shallow breathing during our waking hours, and it is only at night that our breath deepens and slows. Shallow breathing during sleep produces a light, unsatisfying sleep; deep breathing provides refreshing sleep. Since you wish to relax in order to access your qi, your breathing will probably need to be slowed.

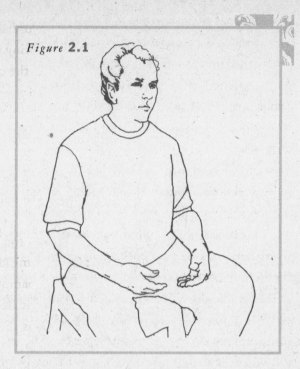

Figure **2.1**

Do not be anxious about accessing your qi. Everybody quickly gets the hang of it.

If it is possible for you to enjoy your breathing during this exercise, that would be ideal. It may be necessary to use your imagination or to rely on your memory to provide you with the sensation of truly pleasurable breathing. Picture or remember yourself in a remote environment of pristine natural beauty, and imagine/recall the pleasure of your first few breaths of clean, cool air. Or, quite the opposite, imagine yourself fleeing from a smoke-filled room, and the dramatic pleasure you take from drawing a few breaths of clean air. If you can enjoy the sensual pleasure of deep, slow breathing, you will quickly access and concentrate your qi.

Do not overdo your deep breathing to the point where you feel light-headed or uncomfortable. What is important is to be aware of your breath and to breathe comfortably.

When you feel relaxed in your mind and upper body, you are ready to begin.

Basic Procedure

With your eyes open, raise your hands, palms facing each other, to the level of your mouth. Your hands should be about six inches apart, and about six inches away from your mouth. If your upper body is relaxed, your hands will assume a natural curve, and your elbows will be turned outward and pointing downward (see Figure 2.2).

It is time to visualize your breath and the qi it will, literally, inspire. Imagine that your breath is a white vapor, the way you would see it come out of your mouth on a cold day.

Exhaling through your mouth, send a slow, steady stream of white vapor between your hands.

Feel the cool vapor fill the space between your palms and fingers. As you continue to exhale slowly, you should be able to see the vapor coalescing into a white ball between your palms. It looks as if you are holding a small round cloud between your hands.

Move your hands in order to play with the white ball. Move them slowly and gently back and forth, up and down, all the time keeping the white ball between your hands. The ball will change its shape as you manipulate it, expanding and contracting to conform with the movement of your hands. Keep exhaling lightly between your palms so that your physical sensation confirms the white cloud's changing shape (see Figure 2.3a).

In about twenty to thirty seconds, your hands will begin to feel an attraction for each other, something like a weak magnetic pull. As you watch your hands moving back and forth, and feel this attraction, you will see that your hands are more and more drawn together naturally. As the distance between your hands diminishes, so does the size of the white ball. Soon your hands will have a strong desire to meet, palms pressing together, but do not let them touch until the feeling of attraction is quite strong (see Figure 2.3b).

When the attraction has grown strong, let your palms come together slowly. As your palms gently meet, the white vapor will be pushed upward where it will hover above your fingertips.

Begin breathing slowly through your nose.

You should now look as if you are praying with your eyes open (see Figure 2.4). Your fingertips and the heels of your palms will be touching. It is not necessary to flatten your palms together. The more relaxed your hands, the faster you will access qi.

Consider your shoulders. Are they tense? Are they raised up high? If so, let them relax by dropping them gently. Your hands will then be at the level of your chest, fingers pointing away from you.

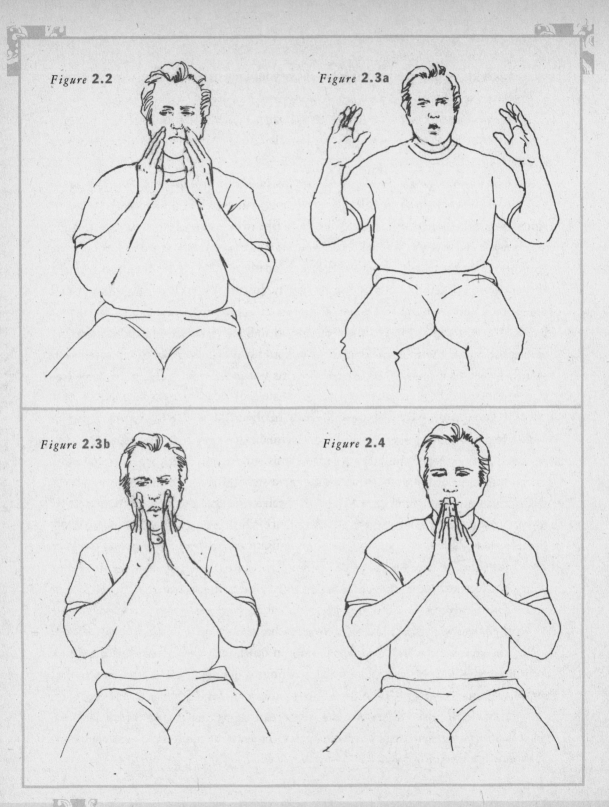

Figure **2.2**

Figure **2.3a**

Figure **2.3b**

Figure **2.4**

Look at the white vapor hovering above your fingertips, and then close your eyes gently (see Figure 2.5, page 30).

Inhale the white vapor through all ten fingertips.

This means that you will, of course, inhale through your nose. However, you will see the white vapor enter into your fingertips. As you inhale, you will feel the vapor coming down your fingers, through your palms, and entering your forearms. The white vapor will go as far as your elbows, at which point you will exhale and watch the vapor retrace its steps until it exits from your fingertips to hover above them once more.

Try to feel the vapor/breath entering and leaving through your hands.

It is neither necessary nor helpful to be anatomically correct when you imagine the course your breath takes through your body. Just think/imagine it happening, and you will feel it as it goes in and out of you.

Your breathing should be rhythmic and unforced. Find a comfortable rhythm and stick to it. By the seventh breath, you should be feeling the white vapor entering your hands as cool air and leaving your body as warm air.

Once you have become aware of this inhale/cool-exhale/warm phenomenon, you will feel your palms begin to tingle slightly in about thirty to sixty seconds. As you continue with your steady breathing and visualization, the tingling sensation will spread to your fingers. Soon, both of your hands will be warm and tingling.

When this occurs, you will be aware of a steady stream of force or energy flowing out of your fingertips. This stream is unrelated to the rhythm of your breath. It does not stop when you inhale and recommence when you exhale. The outward flow seems to have a life of its own and may even pulsate with a rhythm different from your breathing rhythm.

You have accessed your qi.

The qi will continue to flow out of you at a steady pace, regardless of how vigorously you exhale. Many novices, thinking that the force of exhalation controls the force of the qi, push and strain their breath in order to achieve "maximum" flow. In fact, nothing could be further from the workings of qi. The more rhythmic, natural, and relaxed the breathing, the better the outflow of qi.

Having hit your stride, continue your breathing and awareness of the qi leaving your hands for another two or three minutes. This exercise provides so much release from tension and feels so good that many people will keep at it for as long as ten minutes.

It is now time to conclude the procedure.

When you are ready to end this exercise, compress your breath as follows: Raising your head, inhale deeply through your nose, hold the breath a moment, and then with your mouth closed, produce a strong noise in your throat for two seconds. Your breath will now be compressed within your chest, and you will feel tension in your chest, particularly in your solar plexus.

Exhale slowly through your mouth, opening your eyes gradually as you do so.

As your eyes open and your chest relaxes, let your hands fall naturally and slowly back down to your lap.

You have accessed your qi and concentrated it in your solar plexus. You are now ready to transmit qi, either to yourself or to someone else for the purpose of health.

The entire procedure should have taken less than eight minutes.

Once you have grown familiar with, and confident about, this procedure, you may wish to shorten it. Most people stop visualizing the white vapor as the first step. Having experienced the existence of qi and its relation to breathing, the white vapor no longer plays a useful role in accessing qi.

Next, the amount of time it takes between commencing the exercise and having the palms meet usually decreases to about twenty to thirty seconds. The more you practice, the quicker and stronger the attraction between your hands. Nor is it necessary to visualize the flow of breath as far as the elbows. You may simply wish to keep the breath within the palms of your hands and feel them "swell" with air.

However you choose to modify the procedure to suit your own sensibilities, never forget to check for tension in your upper body before beginning, and never forget to keep your breathing steady and gentle.

Intermediate Procedure

The object of this procedure is to create and maintain a breathing connection between the hands and the lower spine.

Seat yourself as you would for the Basic Procedure, and breathe comfortably through your nose.

Be aware of tension in your upper body, particularly in the region of the solar plexus. If you feel a tightness, change the direction you are facing until you find a direction in which you are relaxed.

Raise your hands to the level of your eyes, and place your palms together. Your thumbs should be pointing to the bridge of your nose or between your eyes (see Figure 2.6). Your shoulders will be high, and you will feel tension throughout your upper body.

Take a deep breath through your nose, and, exhaling powerfully, let your shoulders suddenly drop. Your "praying" hands should fall to a position in front of your breastbone or solar plexus. Your upper body will now be completely relaxed. Your fingers will probably be pointing outward (see Figure 2.7).

Close your eyes slowly. Raising your head, inhale deeply through your nose, hold the breath a moment, and then with your mouth closed, produce a strong noise in your throat for two seconds. Your breath will now be compressed within your chest, and you will feel tension in your solar plexus.

Exhale slowly through your hands, your breath beginning at the heels of the palms and moving upward and out through the fingertips.

When first attempting this exercise, it may be a help to return to visualizing your breath as white vapor. It will be clustered and swirling at the bottom of your hands, and then flowing out through your fingertips to reenter when you inhale.

When you feel comfortable with your breathing, imagine your breath passing through your hands and down into the *small of your back.* Do not attempt to have the breath follow an anatomically correct route. It does not matter how the breath gets to the small of the back just as long as it gets there.

The small of the back is located just above the pelvic girdle and is the home of the third and fourth lumbar vertebrae (L3, L4). L3 is located directly behind the navel, although this is not always a helpful hint when trying to find it on yourself. What is easier to locate is L4. Place your hands on your hips. Move your hands slowly upward until they come to the top of your pelvis. Now trace a line from the top of your pelvis to the small of your back, and your thumbs will stop at L4 (see Figure 2.8). This is the area where you should direct your breath.

Direct your breath to that area on your inhalation, let it collect at that spot, and

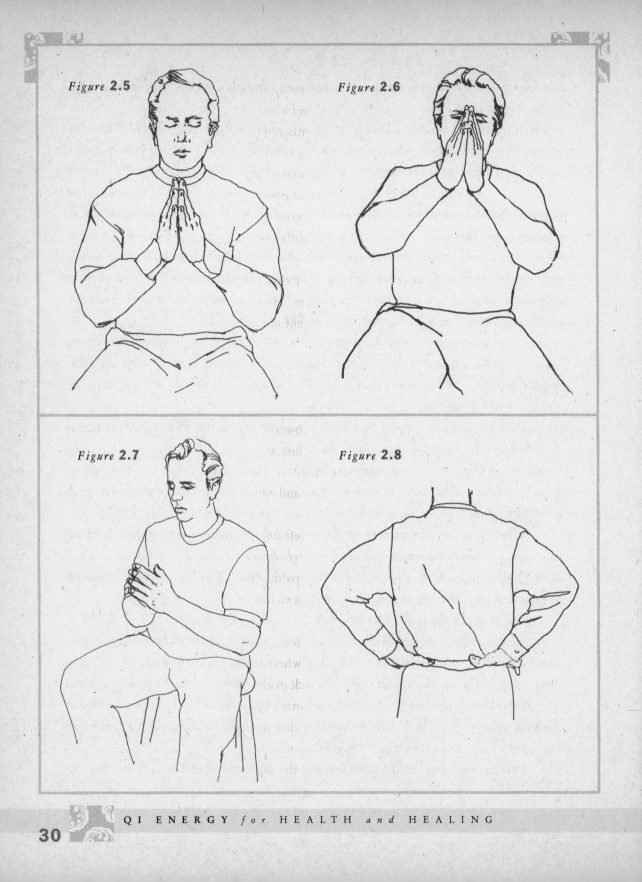

Figure **2.5**

Figure **2.6**

Figure **2.7**

Figure **2.8**

then slowly rise out through your body into your hands and fingers as you exhale. At the beginning of this exercise, many people feel a cool or even cold sensation when the breath collects at L3 and L4. I have seen a number of people actually shiver as they did the exercise. However, after about six or seven breaths, you will feel the vertebrae expand and contract as if they were breathing instead of your lungs. The cold sensation will leave you and will be replaced by a band of pleasant warmth around your midriff. Soon your palms and fingers will tingle, and your qi will begin its wavelike flow out of your hands. Continue your breathing for another two or three minutes, then end the exercise as you did in the Basic Procedure.

This exercise is faster and more efficient than the previous exercise. Further, it produces a sense of full mind/body relaxation. However, you may require a certain amount of trial and error before feeling confident of mastering the technique.

Advanced Procedure

The object of this procedure is to produce a powerful circularity of breath.

This technique follows the same procedure as the Intermediate Procedure until it comes time for the first exhalation.

When you have swallowed your breath and compressed it, *exhale through the fingers of your left hand.*

Imagine the white vapor leaving your left fingertips and hovering above them. *Now inhale the vapor through the fingers of your right hand.*

The white vapor will enter your right palm down to the heel, and then move into the heel of your left palm where it will ascend up and out of your fingers.

You have created a circularity of breath.

After a half dozen breaths, you should feel the breath almost swirling through your right hand, passing into your left hand where the heels of the palms touch, and then shooting out of that hand to be drawn back in again by your right hand, and so on.

The swirling sensation will be accompanied by a warming and tingling of your hands, at which point your qi will begin flowing strongly and effortlessly. Continue breathing in this way for another two or three minutes.

You may end the exercise as you would the Basic Procedure.

Paired Technique

Two people are sitting or standing close together, facing each other. Each person has his or her *right palm down* and *left palm up*. Place your right hand lightly on the other person's left hand (see Figure 2.9).

Close your eyes. On a prearranged signal, each person takes a deep breath, and then simultaneously both of you *exhale through your right hand.* **It is not necessary to synchronize your breathing after this until you end the exercise.**

Do not think about inhaling, only exhaling.

In this exercise, the right hand is active and the left hand is passive. You should soon feel the breath entering your left hand and leaving your right hand in a circular motion. Both hands will grow warm, and you will have the feeling that energy is passing through your chest as it makes its way from hand to hand.

Once you have this sensation of energy, consciously relax your shoulders, and continue breathing comfortably and rhythmically for another two or three minutes.

One person should end the technique.

"On the count of three, let's take a deep breath, and then, as we slowly exhale, open our eyes and let our hands drop to our laps."

Though I call this a "paired technique," any number of people may participate. I have done this exercise with as many as sixty people at one time. One person is the leader. From three people upward, participants form a circle with their hands out at their sides, right palm down and left palm up. The leader counts to three, at which time each person inhales, compresses the breath, and then exhales through the right hand.

All the breath/energy in the room should be moving in a counterclockwise direction.

Figure **2.9**

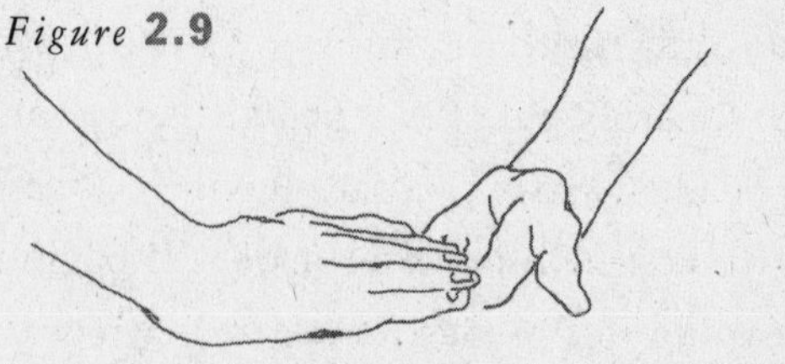

After the initial synchronized breath, each person breathes steadily and naturally at his or her comfortable pace. Since not everyone "warms up" at the same time, it is good to allow more time when accessing qi with a group than you would alone or with a single partner. The leader will end the technique in the same way given above.

The group experience is very interesting for the amount of energy the group generates. Many people report a heady rush like a feeling of being on the verge of levitation during the exercise. It is energizing, relaxing, and fun to produce qi with large numbers of people.

Concentrating and Transmitting Your Qi

The ability to access your qi is the first step to using it for health. It is now time to practice concentrating it in your hands for transmission to yourself or to another. The following exercises are designed to strengthen your qi and sensitize you to the giving and receiving of qi.

Sensitivity requires a state of relaxation. You will have small hope of transmitting your qi effectively if you are brooding whether you should have declared that incidental windfall to the IRS. Place yourself in a restful environment. Background music will help relax you as well.

Access your qi, and as you do so, consciously feel for tension in your shoulders. When the tension has gone and your shoulders are relaxed, your breathing will be deep and you will be ready to transmit qi.

The following exercises are standard procedures regularly performed by all qi practitioners, no matter how proficient. They never grow outmoded nor should you become jaded to their usefulness. In fact, the exercise and training of your qi is one area in which I agree with the Japanese that we should never stray too far from our "beginner's mind."

PAIRED PRACTICE

There needs to be a *giver* and a *receiver* for the following exercises. They should be seated about three feet apart, and the receiver should be at a right angle to the giver. The giver will extend his right arm, the elbow bent at a comfortable angle, and then extend his forefinger and middle finger. The receiver extends her left arm, the elbow bent at a comfortable angle, and then opens her hand to present the giver with a "target." The tableau should look like Figure 2.10.

Technique 1

The giver's fingers should be about six inches from the receiver's palm. The giver may have his eyes open or closed, whichever better aids concentration; however, the receiver should have her eyes closed.

The giver takes a deep breath through the nose, and *exhales through the length of his fingers and out his fingertips*. After two or three such exhalations, qi will begin to flow out of the two fingers. Continue breathing steadily and comfortably.

Remember: the flow of qi is unrelated to the breathing process. It streams out in a continual flow both on the inhalation and on the exhalation. Nor is the flow

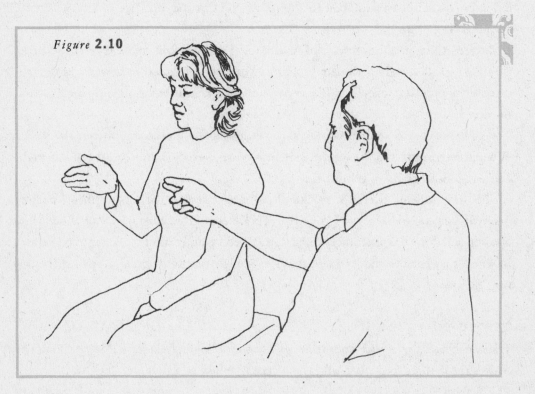

Figure **2.10**

of qi related to the power of the breath. There is no need to force your breath. A relaxed, steady rhythm will maximize the flow of qi.

If you are self-conscious during this exercise, or if you have difficulty concentrating on the qi leaving your fingers, you should talk to yourself internally using precise and concrete expressions to "psych yourself up" or "pump yourself up." You do not have to vocalize. It is more important just to listen to yourself.

"My qi is flowing out of my fingers and into her hand."

"My qi is leaving my body and crossing space to enter her hand."

You may want to be even more positive about what you are doing. For example, "I am sending qi directly from my fingers into the center of her hand, and she is feeling it."

The internal repetition of such phrases is more than just an aid to concentration; it will also strengthen and focus the outflowing qi. When the receiver informs you that she is feeling your qi, you may want to stop repeating your mantra and concentrate on the sensual pleasure of the qi leaving your body.

In under a minute, the receiver should be feeling the qi on her hand. There are many different perceptions of qi, all of them valid. Some people experience a sensation of warmth, others of coolness. Some people report a pulsing, wavelike sensation passing into their palm. The two most common descriptions are of a gentle puff of air against the palm and of a feather lightly tickling the palm.

I once had a highly skeptical and qi-doubting military man as my receiver. He felt a pulsing sensation of waves of warm air brushing against his palm, but insisted that the air conditioner was blowing air on his hands. I turned off the a/c and continued. He next insisted that he was sitting too close to the window, and chinks in the window frame were allowing air to come in. We closed the blinds and moved to the far, windowless corner of the room. He still felt the qi, but this time complained that it was probably coming from the breaths of people around him, practicing like we were. They were banished to the other side of the room. It was a hot Los Angeles summer day, and the hermetically sealed room where ten people held their breath and only two people continued breathing quickly turned into an oven. It was only after all twelve of us were sweating uncomfortably and his hand, now wet with perspiration, still felt the original wavelike sensation, that he admitted the existence of qi.

"I just wanted to make sure," he said, in a burst of understatement.

If, on the other hand, the receiver does not feel your qi, do not be disappointed. It could mean one of two things. One is that you are not concentrating enough, in which case try accessing your qi again. The other is that the receiver is not sensitive enough to have an awareness of the qi, in which case you should have her receive with her right hand from your left hand.

Let us assume that the receiver is feeling the qi in both left and right hands, and that you feel comfortable sending it with either hand. It is now time to switch roles and attempt to feel her qi.

Once you have given and received qi, you and your partner should describe the sensation of qi. This will help you understand the nature of your own qi, and it is of interest to compare the qi you feel from others with the descriptions of your own qi given by others. Words such as *strong, faint, cool, hot, intense, penetrating, diffuse, tranquil,* and *stimulating* are commonly used to describe the sensation of qi.

It is important, while training, for the receiver to inform the giver of any change in the intensity or sensation of qi. The most effective qi for health is that which flows in a steady stream, and receiver feedback will provide the giver with useful information about his projection of qi.

When the receiver senses your qi from six inches away, draw your hand back to eight inches, and then ten inches. If the receiver still feels your qi strongly and steadily, it is time to end the exercise. For beginners, it is customary to spend at least three minutes on each hand. However, feel free to end the exercise whenever you like.

Never end the transmission of qi on an inhalation. Always inhale through your nose, and then, exhaling slowly, gently lower your hand to your lap.

If you and your partner are both able to project your qi strongly and steadily at a distance of ten inches, it is time to move on to the next exercise. If either of you has difficulty sensing the flow of qi, try again. The next exercise requires more heightened sensitivity.

Technique 2

The giver and receiver are seated just as they are in the previous exercise.

The giver will keep his eyes open, but the receiver must have her eyes closed.

QI ENERGY *for* HEALTH *and* HEALING

The giver projects his qi with delicacy and precision by aiming his fingers at a certain point of the receiver's hand from a distance of six inches. It may be the base of the thumb, the exact center of the palm, the tip of the ring finger, or the base of the middle finger, for example.

The giver should be repeating to himself exactly where he is aiming his qi.

"I am sending qi from my fingers into her palm at the base of her forefinger."

The receiver should begin feeling the concentrated qi after about thirty seconds to a minute, at which point she should tell the giver where he is aiming. The receiver may or may not be correct; in either case, aim at a different part of the hand. Try three of four different points.

Technique 3

The face is also a sensitive area to practice on, particularly the eyes, nose, and lips.

The giver and receiver sit facing each other. The giver will keep his eyes open, and the receiver will keep her eyes closed. As in the former exercise, aim your qi as precisely as possible to a spot on the face: between the eyes, the tip of the nose, the middle of the upper lip, or the center of the left eyelid, for example.

Technique 4

This last exercise is quite difficult and requires a high degree of sensitivity on the part of the receiver. However, the results are quite interesting and well worth the effort involved. I do not recommend you attempt this exercise until you feel comfortable with accessing and transmitting your qi.

The giver will write a number on the palm of the receiver.

The giving must be done very slowly and steadily, and the receiver must be very relaxed and focusing concentration on her palm. The giver's fingertip will be at a distance of four to six inches from the receiver's palm. The giver will slowly write a number in the air, all the time intending the qi to trace the number on the receiver's palm. The giver should imagine drawing the number directly on the skin of the receiver's palm. With regular practice, you should be able to "draw and read" numbers (letters are much more difficult) on the palm.

This exercise takes a little more time and effort than the preceding exercises. Do not spend more than ten minutes on the exercise. If you are unable to read the numbers in that amount of time, try again another day.

If you are able to draw and read numbers with both hands at a distance of ten inches, you are able to access your qi using the advanced method and are able to transmit qi for health with confidence.

Remember: the ability to read qi is as important as the ability to project it.

Relaxing the Mind/Body Unity

This solitary exercise is the most difficult of all qi exercises. It is also the most rewarding. The goal is the relaxation of the spine, and from there, the relaxation of the unity of mind/body.

I recommend that this exercise be done sitting, preferably on a firm seat. Both feet should be planted firmly on the floor, and the back should be straight and not leaning against anything. Your head should be resting comfortably on top of your neck, and not lolling to the front or sides. Your hands should be wherever they feel most comfortable. **Remember: by raising your arms, you shorten/tense your spine.** Your arms should be at your sides or on your lap with your shoulders relaxed in order to achieve maximum spine length/relaxation.

Imagine that your spinal cord is a hollow tube connecting the base of your spine with the crown of your head. Be conscious of the spot where your spine meets the seat. Then take two fingers and touch the crown of your head (see Figure 2.11). When location of that point and the sensation of touching that point feel familiar to you, lower your arms and gently close your eyes.

Inhale deeply through your nose, swallow the breath, and then exhale slowly through your nose. Feel your shoulders drop and your upper body relax.

On your next breath, *inhale through the point you have felt on the crown of your head.* To help you do this, you may visualize a nebulous white vapor hovering above that spot. When you inhale through the crown, the white vapor is sucked into your head at that point, and the inside of your head suddenly feels refreshingly cool. Now imagine the white vapor traveling down the length of the hollow tube that is your spine.

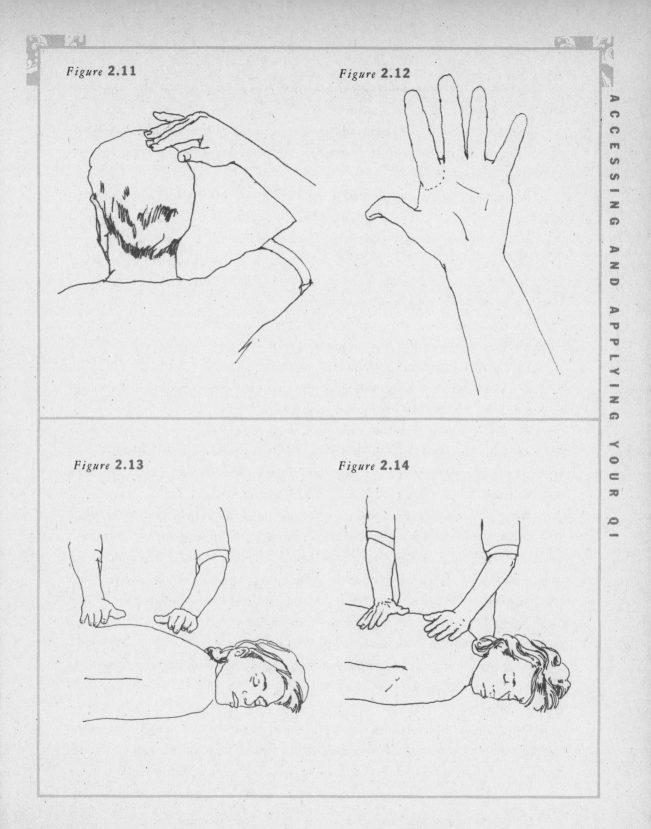

Figure **2.11**

Figure **2.12**

Figure **2.13**

Figure **2.14**

Be aware of your spine ending at the point where it meets the seat. Your breath can go no further than this.

When the white vapor reaches this terminus, it leaves the hollow tube and fills the large cavity where the base of your spine meets the seat. In other words, you are now sitting on your breath.

When you exhale, imagine this diffuse white vapor being sucked up into the hollow tube and moving slowly upward until it leaves the top of your head through the crown. The vapor will hover over that point until you inhale again.

On your next inhalation, feel the coolness of the white vapor and "see" it travel down the length of your spine. Feel the coolness collect in the cavity at the base of your spine as you "watch" the vapor fill that cavity.

After two or three more such breaths, the base of your spine will feel cool; at the same time, however, you may begin sweating from the scalp or forehead.

Do not be alarmed—this is an ideal reaction.

Continue your breathing, and enjoy the rhythm of your breathing, the steady, endless flow of air moving up and down your spine.

For those who have attained a facility with this exercise:

Your spinal cord is still a hollow tube, but it is a tube made of individual connecting tubes called vertebrae. You may think of a vertical train with a long row of cars creating a single line. The exact number of vertebrae is unimportant for this exercise. What is important is to imagine/visualize the breath passing from vertebra to vertebra.

Imagine you are looking at your body from the side, in silhouette. You see your spinal cord running from the base of your skull to the seat. Visualize the white vapor passing slowly from vertebra to vertebra. After a couple of breaths, you will feel your spinal cord relax. Do not be surprised if you suddenly feel light-headed or weightless. Some people feel as if they are rising upward off their seat.

Do not be alarmed. There has never been a verified levitation sighting.

Your overall feeling of lightness aside, you should not be feeling the existence of any part of your anatomy other than what lies between the crown of your head and the seat of your pants.

This exercise has a dual purpose: relaxation and sensitization. There is, therefore, no time limit on doing this exercise. When you wish to end the exercise, exhale through the crown of your head, and imagine the white vapor dispersing into thin air.

Next, inhale consciously through your nose, swallow the breath, exhale slowly through your mouth, and slowly open your eyes.

This exercise is particularly challenging, but its rewards are commensurate with its degree of difficulty. It will become a valuable relaxation tool. You have only to manage to be alone for five minutes, and this brief and effective exercise will provide the physical relaxation and mental clarity to carry on with whatever you need to do.

In addition, many people report significant and immediate relief from lower backache by doing this exercise.

Qi for Pets

The qi you project mirrors your current emotional state. If you are agitated about finances or disappointed in love, your qi will have those qualities, and you are unlikely to produce soothing or healing effects when transmitting your qi. Your qi will be hesitant, tentative, and perhaps even agitated.

On the other hand, should you feel on top of the world, relaxed, happy, and satisfied, your qi will produce highly effective results in a short amount of time. In other words, qi produced by worry, tension, or agitation will likely produce similar effects in others, while qi produced through relaxation and benevolence will produce a soothing and tranquilizing effect that is the first step to healing.

The trouble is that, with the hustle and bustle and tension in our daily lives, we are hardly aware of our current emotional state. Certainly, we do not have a clear and focused awareness of the degree of tension we are carrying within us. A simple but trying forty-minute car ride from home to office can produce an emotional state that colors the rest of the day. Added to this is the desensitization that comes from living in artificially controlled environments and enjoying an unvarying diet that bears no relation to the change of the seasons. No wonder that we humans have but a meager awareness of the strength, texture, and feel of our qi at any given moment. Other animals, however, are extremely sensitive to the texture of qi and will give us an immediate and unequivocal response to the qi we project. What follows is an interesting approach to gauging your qi and to bringing out the Saint Francis in you.

Let us assume you have a pet. If you do not, you probably know someone who has, and who would be happy to let you spend a few minutes with it. The following exercise can be done with either a dog or a cat. I have found cats respond more quickly and demonstrably than dogs, so for the purpose of my example, I will use a cat.

Access your qi and, having done so, look for your cat. Chances are it will be sleeping on that one piece of furniture you are forever shooing it from. Do not be annoyed, or the experiment will be doomed to failure.

Remember: cats were placed on Earth to test our patience and qualifications for sainthood.

Sit in a comfortable position on a couch or in an easy chair . . . anywhere that you and the cat can feel relaxed together. You may be listening to soothing music or watching TV. If possible, keep your back straight, but this is not absolutely necessary. It is more important to have both you and the cat resting comfortably.

Place the cat on your lap. Give it a minute to situate itself and fall into that twilight world of restful cat life. Place one hand (the right hand if possible) on the cat's spine. Your palm may be either horizontal or vertical to the spine, whichever suits your posture. I have found the horizontal position more natural and more comfortable to maintain. Try to keep your hand resting lightly and away from the cat's head.

Look at your hand on the cat's spine for a moment. Then, inhaling quietly through your nose, exhale through the palm of your hand and into the spine of the cat.

There is no need for any visualization. Simply feel your breath leave your hand and enter the spine of the cat. Your qi will be flowing out steadily into the creature's body. Maintain a steady, comfortable rhythm of breathing.

By your third breath, the cat will be aware of your qi. Most cats respond by the second breath and indicate this by a large twitch. Now comes the test.

If your qi is agitated or tentative or abrupt, the cat will react at once, sometimes by bristling and even snarling. Fur standing on end is a sign of extreme displeasure. Most cats react to a disturbance in the qi with a small shriek, jump off your lap, and rush out of the room.

The cat's reaction to soothing and steady qi is the complete opposite. It will begin to purr and lapse into an apparent kitty coma. At this point, you will probably spend the next ten minutes considering how to extricate yourself without disturbing this picture of Perfect Bliss.

The cat's reaction to your qi is in no way an evaluation of the general properties of your qi. It is an indication of your present mood or state of mind. You may try the exercise six days in a row and get a different reaction each day.

My cat, Basil, and I do qi training almost every night before bed. He is now a veteran of the qi experience and swings between being a qi junkie and a qi connoisseur: some nights he just needs a fix, and other nights he evaluates qi critically. Because he reacts with violent displeasure to any disturbance in my qi, I put myself into a relaxed and bonhomous state of mind before putting hands on him. I find that I cannot watch the late news and satisfy Basil. The news is usually too disturbing. So, listening to music, I put qi into Basil's spine, which soothes both of us, and we sleep the better for it.

A skilled but eccentric gentleman with whom I studied qi in Japan claimed to practice on his fish. He had a small pond with koi (carp) in his garden. He would place his hand under water and send qi throughout the pond, giving each fish a pretty good dose. He maintained that the qi tranquilized them and that they would swim in slow ecstasy. I never witnessed this and only put it forward for future experimentation. My own experience with fish was quite the opposite.

It happened when our son was in preschool. We went to his school carnival, and I lost sight of him in the crush for about a minute. During which time, he succeeded in achieving the unthinkable: he won a living prize at a rather difficult pitch-and-toss event. This prize was a tiny goldfish in a small plastic bag with about enough water in it to wiggle its wee tail. This prize package had been standing in 106-degree sunlight most of the day, and the fish looked poached. Seeing the shock and sadness in my eyes, the prize giver sought to console me.

"Don't worry," said the fish lady, "these fish are guaranteed to die within three days."

Our son named the fish Goofy, declared he loved it more than anything in the world, and brought it into the house to live with him forever.

We got Goofy a little fishbowl and a lot of fresh water. On the third morning of Goofy's arrival, our son woke us to say that Goofy had stopped swimming and was sleeping on his side at the bottom of the fishbowl. Sure enough, Goofy was looking like a flounder that had just suffered a coronary. I prodded him, he seemed dead, and I went to get the net to scoop him out and inter his remains in the toilet.

"Oh, do something, Mama, do something," our son implored my wife.

Rising to the drama of the moment, she stuck her finger in the fishbowl, aimed at the lifeless Goofy, and began sending qi for all she was worth. I cupped the bowl with both hands, and felt her qi swirling in the water. Now comes the amazing part.

Goofy remained inert for at least a minute. My wife and I were giving up hope when all of a sudden *he swam straight up to the top of the tank and leapt out of the water like a rocket!*

That fish leapt and dove and swam in circles like a hooked marlin. There was nothing tranquil or mellow about his reaction. He swam to the side of the fishbowl and stared at my wife as if memorizing every line on her face.

Goofy returned from the dead by means of qi, I am sure of it. He returned (or turned out to be) a female, and so our son, being a Francophile, renamed her Gaufée.

Gaufée is still alive and well years later, about six inches long with a beautiful gossamer tail and fins. My wife has only to enter the room for Gaufée to swim to the side of the bowl and stare out at her. She then leaps out of the water, my wife shoots her a little qi, and she is happy in her tank the rest of the day, a very animated fish.

In short, because your pets are living creatures, they possess the same features of qi that you do. You should feel no hesitation to use your qi for the ongoing health of your pets, to get them over an illness, or to help them heal after an accident or surgical procedure.

Applying Your Qi

GENEROSITY OF SPIRIT

There is a unity of intention and the effective flow of qi. The most potent qi is that which is generated and guided by a generosity of spirit. As I wrote earlier, the satisfaction one takes in life does not imply a self-seeking hedonism. Regard for others is central to the efficacy of healing qi. In the words of William Blake, "The most sublime act is to set another before you."

You cannot kill a person with qi. You can wish someone dead as you transmit your qi, but qi will not make your wish come true. At worst, you will make the person feel anxious or nauseated. More probably, your qi will not be the least effective simply because it does not blend with the qi of the receiver. Just as it is next to impossible to transmit qi successfully to a mean-spirited person, so it is unthinkable that a mean-spirited person can generate effective healing qi.

On the other hand, wishing someone well as you transmit qi will work toward making him or her well. To have a loving thought in mind as you give qi enlarges and fortifies your qi.

You may also have a conscious intention of healing a specific ailment or treating a specific wound or blow. Intention is not the be-all and end-all of healing qi, but no amount of technical expertise or finesse can make up for a lack of good intention and generosity of spirit.

I never begin to give qi treatment without thinking of a loved person, living or dead, whose approval energizes me. I conjure up his or her face when I do my warm-up exercises to access my qi, and I imagine us breathing together. I feel a rhythmic union with the person and dedicate my day's work to that person. I work for that person's approval by helping others on their behalf. Thus, I set out to do a day's work with good intentions and a generosity of spirit.

APPLYING QI

The application of qi depends on the size and location of the area to be treated. There are three fundamental ways of giving qi: through the fingers, through the hands, and through the circular area at the base of the forefinger.

Touch the base of your forefinger and you will feel a round, prominent bone. This bone is the center of a small circular area that is highly effective for transmitting qi (see Figure 2.12, page 39). In traditional Japanese martial arts, it is known as "the fourth point" and, when applied effectively, creates a lot of pain. In traditional Japanese healing arts, it is called "the tranquil point" and, when applied effectively, alleviates pain. I like to refer to this point as the "heart" of the hand for the transmission of healing qi.

Remember: whenever you transmit qi, be sure to begin and end on an exhalation.

When you begin to give qi, the spot that is receiving it will begin to feel warm under your fingers in less than a minute. It may even feel as if, rather than your giving it the qi, the spot is taking the qi from you. The sensation is as if your qi is being quickly sucked out of your fingers or hands.

In a minute or two, the sensation of warmth will reach its peak and then plateau. Once the plateau has been reached, the area will begin to cool down. In another minute, it may actually feel cold to the touch. This means that the spot has absorbed all the qi it can, and it is pointless to try to force more qi into it. It would be like adding water to a saturated sponge. Remove your fingers on an exhalation, and wait at least an hour before attempting to give qi to the same spot.

Qi is not magic. The giving and receiving of qi involves physiological processes. Therefore, rather than "go for the home run" and attempt to eliminate pain at a single go, attempt to hit a single or a double, meaning the alleviation of pain. The qi will continue to work at the cellular level after you have removed your hands, and the pain may later be eliminated.

Remember: healing with qi is like cooking with microwaves—the process continues even after the current is turned off.

RELAXATION

Do not hesitate to try to apply your qi from the moment you are able to access it. You do not have to pass a series of exams in order to apply your qi. The training exercises given above should be regularly practiced and repeated. A familiarity and facility with those exercises will strengthen and refine your qi, and will also relax and sensitize your body. Accessing your qi results in a state of relaxation that also makes you highly susceptible to receiving qi. However, the average recipient of your qi (spouse, child, parent, or friend, for example) does not practice any relaxation technique before receiving your qi. *Therefore, relaxing the receiver is essential for the effective transmission of your qi.*

No two people relax in the same way. Some people will scream at you through clenched teeth, "I am relaxed dammit!" Others will think a happy thought and lapse into a relaxed reverie. Certainly, before any qi treatment, it is best to try to induce a state of repose. *The procedures that follow should be used at the start of any qi session.* They are neither time consuming, nor tedious to give or receive. To abbreviate or even by-pass a relaxation procedure will usually result in the failure to transmit qi effectively.

You Relax Your Receiver

The receiver should lie facedown with his arms alongside his body. The spine is at its longest and most relaxed when the arms are by the body's side. (Pregnant women whose pregnancy is "showing" should not lie in the prone position. For women in the early stage of pregnancy, if you are able to sleep on your stomach, you are able to do this exercise. Techniques for relaxing a pregnant woman will be given in Chapter 5.)

The receiver's head should be facing right, resting on the left cheek.

The giver will be at the receiver's left, meaning that the giver's right hand will be at the receiver's lower back, and the left hand will be at the head.

In Japan, this exercise is performed on the floor, with the giver sitting on her knees in the classical Japanese position known as *seiza.* I do not recommend this position except for the truly initiated or the pain-loving.

For those with access to a massage table, the giver should be standing. Massage tables equipped with face cradles make this exercise particularly relaxing for the receiver, as the neck is straight rather than turned to the right.

Most people will probably use a bed for the procedure. The receiver will be lying at the left edge of the bed, and the giver will be seated on a chair or low stool by the side of the bed at about the same height as the receiver.

When both parties are comfortable, the giver tells the receiver to close his eyes. The giver keeps her eyes open throughout the course of this procedure.

With your hands lying lightly in your lap, observe the breath of the receiver. Is it deep and slow? Is it rapid and shallow? How far down into the body does the breath go? A really deep, refreshing breath will cause the backside to rise up, while a shallow breath will be confined to the area of the lungs. Chances are that the breathing will tend toward the rapid and shallow.

Having observed his breathing, raise your hands above the receiver's spine, palms down. You will look like a concert pianist about to launch into a solo (see Figure 2.13, page 39).

The left hand should be four to six inches below the base of the neck, and the right hand will be just above the waistline.

With your hands about three inches above the receiver's spine, and still observing his breathing, *inhale deeply through your nose and exhale through the palms of your hands, intending to send qi from your whole hand into the receiver's spine.*

You may want to think about what you are doing.

"I am sending qi from my hands into his spine. I am relaxing his spine and deepening his breathing by means of my qi" . . . or some such message.

As you grow more confident, turn off the message and forget about your own breathing. Just breathe comfortably and naturally, and feel the flow of qi leaving your hands. Your breathing will almost certainly be slower and deeper than the receiver's.

When you observe that the receiver is at the peak of his inhalation, gently lower your hands to lie on the receiver's spine at the points indicated earlier (see Figure 2.14, page 39). Feel your hands riding on his back, going up and down in sync with his breathing.

Synchronize one of your exhalations with one of the receiver's.

As you see and feel the receiver begin to exhale, exhale together with him, and send qi from your palms directly into his spine. There is no need to synchronize the speed of your exhalation, nor is there any need to attempt synchronized breathing. Breathe at a comfortable and steady pace, regardless of the speed of the receiver's breathing.

You are breathing to stay alive, not to transmit qi. The qi will be flowing out steadily on its own.

Again, for those trying this for the first or second time, an internal "mantra" of positive thought will be an aid to your effort.

"Qi is coming out of my hands all the time."

"I am relaxing his spine by sending qi into it."

In less than a minute, the receiver's breath should have slowed and deepened.

———

When you notice this, continue applying your qi for another thirty seconds to a minute, paying particular attention to the rhythm of the receiver's breath.

To end the procedure, synchronize an exhalation with the receiver. When his lungs are fully inflated, begin your exhalation to coincide with his.

Think consciously that your qi is flowing out of your palms and into his spine.

When you run out of breath, gently lift both hands off the receiver's back as you begin your inhalation. Place your hands comfortably on your lap.

The receiver's mind and body are now susceptible to qi treatment.

As you acquire expertise and confidence in the application of qi, you will be able to relax an individual in less than a minute. Of course, the longer you apply qi, the more profound the relaxation will be. The application of qi to the spine is a wonderful tool to relaxing the body and clearing the mind, which in itself is of great benefit to a tense or highly stressed individual.

A HELLO TO ARMS

People love having their upper arm held. I am not sure why this is so, but I conjecture that the feeling instills a sense of security and protection. In the case of a righty, grasp the right upper arm, and for a lefty, the left upper arm. The person can be seated or lying on her back.

Using both hands in the shape of a ring, grasp the subject's upper arm and apply gentle, steady pressure for thirty seconds (see Figure 2.15). Release the pressure while keeping your hands in place.

Exhale through the palms of your hands, sending qi into the arm.

Squeeze gently but firmly as

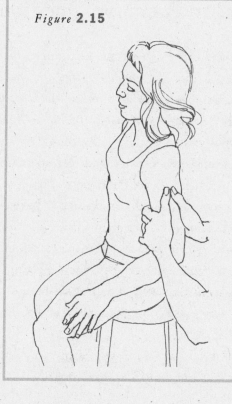

Figure **2.15**

you did before, this time feeling the qi flow out of your hands. Apply pressure for thirty seconds. Release the pressure while keeping your hands in place. Wait ten seconds. Repeat the procedure twice more.

Feel free to move your "ring" up and down the subject's arm. You can grasp from the armpit down to the elbow. In fact, some spots will relax the subject better than others. I like my arm held just above the elbow, while most people prefer to have their arm held higher up.

After your first application of qi, you will see that the subject's shoulders will drop or slope downward. The person is now relaxed.

Remove your "ring" from the subject's arm on an exhalation.

Sending qi through your hands will enhance the relaxation process, but it is not necessary to do so. Simply holding the arm will produce the desired effect.

The Most Common Question

Most people think that we have a limited amount of energy, which, if depleted, will lead to exhaustion, fatigue, and illness. It is as if energy is like blood: should we lose any, it takes time and rest to restore the loss. This leads them to ask me, "Don't you get really tired after you give a treatment? Don't you have to rest between patients? Do you just zonk out when you go home after work?"

The answers are *no, no,* and *no,* respectively.

The truth is quite the opposite. Energy creates and re-creates itself. If you remember your childhood, you seemed to have boundless energy, enthusiasm, and exuberance. As an adult, when something interests or intrigues you, you can stick to it effortlessly and time passes faster than you would wish.

I find that a one-hour business meeting leaves me enervated and feeling as if I had just spent six weeks in hell. A six-hour day of giving qi treatments, on the other hand, leaves me feeling exhilarated and satisfied, and I marvel at how quickly the day passed.

When, as a novice, you apply your qi, you may at first feel tired. This indicates that *you are trying too hard.*

All of us beginners put more effort into a procedure than the procedure actually requires. That goes for swinging a tennis racket, using a computer keyboard, playing the saxophone, and giving qi.

You will quickly realize that qi flows out best when it flows out comfortably and rhythmically with a good intention propelling it. And best of all, the more you give, the more you retain.

CHAPTER 3

Our Latent Power

Adapting and Adjusting

There are many benefits to transmitting qi.

1. The transmission of qi to another accelerates the individual's healing powers by stimulating the body's latent energy and physical strength.

2. A healthy individual is one whose body is harmonious in all movement, internal and external. Giving and receiving qi promotes the self-maintenance of that harmony. This self-maintenance is the body's natural adaptive power. The effectiveness of the adaptive power resides in its sensitivity to ceaselessly changing stimuli, and in its speed and strength of response.

3. Giving and receiving qi promotes the effective functioning of the adaptive power. In this way, physical health and mental vigor are restored and maintained.

4. Giving and receiving qi demonstrates to the individual his own adaptive power and guides him in perpetuating self-maintenance.

5. Ultimately, a facility with transmitting qi frees the individual from total reliance on external health care.

Read on to learn more.

How the Body Adapts

You cannot consciously will your heart to stop beating or your stomach to stop functioning. You cannot demand your body to cease processing the elements you put in it, such as polluted air, lite beer, and greasy food. The power of prayer will exert no influence on the quantity of hair you maintain or lose on your head.

On the other hand, the gradual accumulation of negative external influences—say, financial worries, unhappy personal relationships, troubles on the job—*can* cause your heart to stop beating and your stomach to malfunction. You may develop ulcers or suffer a heart attack. Prolonged worry will eventually cause your hair to fall out or lead to constipation.

Your body has reacted to certain stimuli and has suffered for it. The suffering was not sudden and unexpected. It was steady and cumulative. During the "buildup to breakdown," your body sought to protect you from the negative stimuli. It alerted you to your condition by headaches, stiff shoulders, gastric pain, heartburn, sleep disorders, and other means, and in so doing, kept you functioning longer than might be expected. In the end, your body was physically overwhelmed by the constancy and intensity of the mental and physical stress to which it was subjected—or, to put it bluntly, to which you subjected it. What I wish to suggest here is the fact that your body strove to maintain and prolong your health right up until the moment it was overwhelmed.

Then there is the well-known and often cited example of an average man or woman who, at a moment of crisis, performs a "superhuman" feat. The average person could not possibly walk over to a car and lift up its front end. However, there are authenticated stories of an average person seeing someone knocked down by, and pinned under, a car, and running over and lifting the car off the victim. The physiological workings behind this scenario, as in the case of the preceding paragraph, are not as important as the phenomenon itself: the body reacted to certain stimuli in a certain way, this time in a successful, lifesaving way.

What these extreme scenarios demonstrate is the body's latent energy and strength for producing beneficial results, that is, the prolongation of life. This chapter seeks to instruct the reader into the nature of this latent energy and into its use for healing and for maintaining the health of the body.

Let us look more closely at the example of the person who saves a life by lifting up the front end of a car. The body received a stimulus and reacted to that stimulus. To put it another way, the body quickly and efficiently adapted to the sudden event it encountered. It did so naturally, without any conscious thought on the part of the individual. There was simply a reflex response, the impulse to "do good." The nervous system sent out urgent signals, adrenaline and other chemicals were instantly secreted, the lungs took a deep breath, oxygen flowed into the blood cells, and a number of other physiological processes occurred in an instant. With only the intention to save a life, the body's strength momentarily increased a hundredfold, and a life was saved.

This super power was momentary, for it was needed only for a moment. Once the need has been fulfilled, in other words, once the body has done what it has to do (save a life), it readapts to a new situation, a situation that does not require all the adrenaline and muscle power and oxygen it now possesses. The adrenaline and other chemicals must be flushed from the body or they will, with time, turn stale and toxic. The muscles must relax. They will probably be sore from this unexpected exertion. The nervous system must calm itself, the heart rate must slow down, and so on. The organism will readjust itself to its prestimulated status.

This natural behavior to react to stimuli is what I call the body's *adaptive power,* and it is qi that maintains and regulates this power.

The example I have just given is large and dramatic. I do not wish the reader to think that the body's latent power is confined to such macroscopic stimuli. The human body encounters thousands of tiny stimuli daily, some so small we do not even think of them as stimuli. We walk out of our home into the fresh air, and we are met with a different temperature to which we must adapt. We hear loud noises, soft noises, sudden noises that our senses and mind must adapt to if we are to survive the day. We meet people we like and people we dislike, and we react in different ways. We drink too little water and too much coffee. The former must be retained while the latter must be cleansed from our system. We eat some food that we enjoy, and some food whose taste, texture, and composition are so unappetizing that we prefer to think of it as fuel rather than food. The body must overcome its own distaste with the meal to extract some nourishment from it.

Though we take it for granted, it is astonishing how our bodies continually and effectively adapt to each and every one of these internal and external stimuli. The body's obsession with micromanagement makes the most compulsive supervisor look like a slouch. This is the microscopic working of our latent energy, which is roused into action by our natural adaptive power.

The effectiveness of our natural adaptive power resides in our sensitivity to ceaselessly changing stimuli, and in the speed and strength (latent energy) of the body's response.

If your body is invaded by bacteria, the healthy adaptive response is quickly to run a fever in order to burn away the invaders. It is confusing cause and effect to think that bacteria produce fever. We encounter tens of thousands of bacteria daily and never bat an eyelash. However, when the body's ever-vigilant immune system senses a dangerous trespasser, it launches a brief investigation, and then takes appropriate action to repel the intruder. You cannot will your body to take different measures.

If you get a piece of grit in your eye, your body adapts to the discomfort by turning on tears in order to wash the grit away, and the sooner the better. In the same way, your body adapts to an extreme psychological situation by using tears and vocal sounds as cleansing mechanisms. Whether produced by joy or sorrow, tears and sobs release and remove a powerful emotion from the body where, if left pent up, the emotion would lead to physical discomfort or dysfunction.

On a more lighthearted note, you can work yourself into ill health in order to clear your desk in time for your vacation. You may leave for your vacation feeling like something the cat dragged in, but on the morning of the first day of that longed-for vacation, you feel like a million dollars, and your body is more than up to the task of sudden exercise and exertion.

It is qi that promotes the effective functioning of the adaptive power; it

is, therefore, through the working of qi that physical health and mental alertness are maintained and improved.

There is one more thing to be said about our natural adaptive power, and it will be a recurring theme throughout this book that will be enlarged upon later. Our adaptive power responds both micro- and macroscopically to a continuing barrage of stimuli. This may be called *dealing with the present.* On top of all this, as if just dealing with this barrage were not enough, the body is also *dealing with the past and with the future.*

All of the events in our lives occur within a time continuum and, therefore, have a context. Let us return to our car lifter and put that incident in perspective.

Her name is Liz Dunn, and she is a sixty-four-year-old widow living alone. Her late husband was in the military, and died in a work-related accident eight years ago. Her only child, Charles, is forty years old, and lives halfway across the country.

Liz has a part-time job with a barely adequate salary, and so has been financially dependent on her late husband's military benefits. One day, about two weeks before lifting the front end of the car, she received two communications: a letter from the Veterans Administration informing her that her benefits were to be reduced by 12 percent in accordance with their cost-cutting measures; and an air ticket from her son, Charles, with a sweet note inviting her to spend Thanksgiving with him and his family.

The note from the VA sent her into a tizzy of alarm. She lost her appetite and had trouble falling asleep. At work, she found that rather than concentrating on what she was doing, she was thinking about how to economize to make ends meet. Sometimes her chest felt so tight that she could hardly breathe, and that would induce brief weeping that relieved the strain.

At the same time, she looked forward to seeing Charles and his family, though she hated to fly. It was not fear of flying that bothered her. It was the packing and unpacking and sitting around at the airport and having her flight delayed or canceled and the cramped airplane seats, and then waiting endlessly for her baggage at the other end.

From the moment the two communications arrived until the moment Liz saw the traffic victim hit by the car, her body was adapting and adjusting to the past stimulus of her bad financial news and to the future stimulus of her impending plane flight, *all the while adapting and adjusting to present stimuli.*

Her body was attempting to ameliorate the physical stress her tense emotional state had produced so that she could continue to function in daily life. At the same time, her body was adjusting itself to the idea of a three-hour plane flight, so that it would be ready and resilient to make a successful trip when the day came . . .

When suddenly, an event exploded upon Liz's present that called for an instant adjustment. When the person had been saved and she released the car, Liz's body went immediately back to dealing with her past and future adjustments, even as it adapted to the immediate change of events, that is, great physical strength was no longer needed and she had to relax.

Even as the body copes and responds to the present, it deals with the legacy of the past and the promise of the future.

Apart from the unexpected, such as Liz encountered, we never enter into a situation that our bodies have not already prepared for, nor, until there is a decisive conclusion, do we ever stop adjusting to past events. When Liz boards that plane, her body will not play catch-up, but will be fully prepared for the flight. And unless Charles offers to make up the 12 percent pension cut, her Thanksgiving appetite will not improve.

I have just used the words *situation* and *events* to refer to past and future, but there is one more past and future to which the body never ever ceases to adapt: the change of seasons.

Our bodies start to adapt to the oncoming cold of winter from the end of summer, and spring starts manifesting itself within our bodies from the middle of January. We never enter a new season in the mode of a prior season, but always fully adapted to the new season. The adjustment is gradual, so that we have, as it were, one foot in the past and one in the future. The fact that our adjustment is gradual leads people to overlook or ignore its workings, no matter how obvious they might be. The importance of this seasonal adaptation and the harmful consequences of a weak adaptive power to the seasons will be taken up later.

Thus, from the standpoint of our natural adaptive power and all it must do just to keep us functioning, we can imagine a traditional timepiece with large and small wheels and even smaller cogs and gears and tiny teeth that must mesh perfectly to keep the mechanism running smoothly. Yet the intricacy and complexity of our adaptive mechanism is immeasurably greater than that of any man-made machinery. Qi keeps us running and humming along so that the in/external harmony of all our bodily movements is maintained through our natural adaptive power.

Stress and the Flow of Qi

Any idiot can face a crisis—it's this day-to-day living that wears you out.
— ANTON CHEKHOV

Left to its own devices, the human body would self-monitor and self-regulate its flow of qi in order to keep itself at optimum health. It would, all by itself, keep itself as healthy as its innate adaptive power allowed. There are, however, several reasons why this ideal state does not come about. For the purpose of this book, only one reason—the prime reason—need be advanced: stress. Stress is induced by personal and environmental factors. Stress is the main impediment to the healthy functioning of the organism. There is a growing school of medical opinion that believes that stress, together with genetic factors, is at the root of many illnesses, including cancer.

Make a fist. Clench it tight. Feel the muscles bulge in your forearm. Feel the ache in your palm. Now try to brush your teeth. Or drive a car. Or hold a fork. Or sew a button on a shirt. Obviously you can't. And the number of things you can't do in this state is infinitely greater than the number you can.

The "unnatural," excessive tension in the hand is impeding the hand's functions. It is by relaxing the hand that you can comb your hair or type an E-mail. In the same way, stress resulting in physical tension impedes the self-regulating activities of the body, which in turn impairs health. To put it another way, the flow of qi within the body encounters insurmountable obstacles.

The qi that you feel leaving your hands when you do the preceding exercises, and the qi that you feel when you receive qi from another person are the same qi that is continuously coursing through your body. The flow of qi is the body's equivalent of running a virus scan or a disk scan on your computer. The qi is ceaselessly monitoring the body's activities and movements at the micro- and macroscopic levels, and making adjustments where need be. Stress impedes the flow of qi and causes gaps in the monitoring process.

It is as if a technician charged with monitoring the machinery of a large laboratory finds half of the doors inexplicably locked against him as he makes his rounds. When the body is dominated by tension, it loses its chief technician and mechanic, qi. This is when breakdowns in the system occur: headaches, stiff shoulders, backache, poor digestion, sleep disorders, irregular periods, male impotence, skin eruptions, and worse.

A Question of Balance

In twenty-three years of learning and practicing qi medicine, no one has ever said to me, "Dr. Fromm, I am just too damned relaxed. Isn't there anything you can do to put a little tension in my life?" Should I ever meet such a person, I would treat him for narcolepsy.

Our bodies tense when we inhale and relax when we exhale. If it were only as easy as breathing to maintain the balance between tension and relaxation, the health status of most of the world would improve dramatically. Unfortunately, the balance scales of our daily lives are heavily weighted in favor of tension. With tension comes a loss of flexibility and with a loss of flexibility comes an accompanying loss of durability. As I wrote earlier, health is not a matter of strength or "fitness," but a matter of flexibility, both mental and physical. The example I gave above of a clenched fist as a total loss of flexibility was an extreme one, but I frequently treat bodies that have reached that extreme and, even more frequently, encounter bodies that are on their way to becoming that extreme.

One easy way to relax a body and clear a mind of tension is to send qi into the spine. The flow of qi through the spine is a very quick and effective means of relaxation. It may be done alone (see "Relaxing the Mind/Body Unity" on page 38) and it may be done with another (see "You Relax Your Receiver" on page 47).

Though both procedures are excellent means of relaxation, they do not go so far as to restore the equilibrium of tension and relaxation *throughout* the body, including the organs.

The unimpeded flow of qi will restore the body's tension/relaxation equilibrium and arouse its latent powers.

But how to achieve that goal? The answer lies in the working of qi on the extrapyramidal motor system (EMS) and on the autonomic nervous system (ANS).

The Extrapyramidal Motor System and the Autonomic Nervous System

The extrapyramidal motor system and the autonomic nervous system govern all facets of the balance of tension and relaxation within the body. The application of qi to the EMS will trigger a flow of energy throughout that system and throughout the ANS. This energy flow will bypass the central nervous system and transcend thought (conscious behavior). It will sweep away blockages and barriers to the smooth passage of qi. It will remove tension and promote relaxation and will restore the functioning of organs to their original integrity. In Japanese, the exercise promoting the uninhibited flow of qi is called *kiryū*.

Kiryū creates physical anarchy in a way we have not experienced since early childhood. We were then free to respond to the body's demands and express its striving for health any way we liked. We could fart, belch, burp, roll around on the floor, cry, yell and scream, jump and run, giggle uncontrollably—all with impunity. As we aged and learned manners and entered society, we learned to suppress a fart, squelch a belch, curb our physical impulses, and so on. In other words, we repress and suppress all the hundreds of little release mechanisms designed to rid ourselves of tension.

Above all, we feel self-conscious about movement. We join movement classes and dance classes and exercise classes in order to have a safe and approved environment in which to move in a manner different from our "everyday" manner. No one seems to notice that while our minds are in constant motion, our bodies hardly move in proportion in our daily life.

Social conventions state that the fewer our movements, the more well behaved we are. "Children should be seen and not heard." We take pride when our young children do not run around and make noise in a restaurant, but sit with a minimum of movement and talk. "We are good parents," we think, "we have taught our children self-control. Now we can enjoy our meal."

Looked at from your own physiology, stress can "teach" you self-control. Stress can impair the movements of cells, nerves, muscles, and organs so that they sit quietly doing nothing. What you applaud in your children's behavior you look askance at in your body's behavior. Your palate fails to function and you do not enjoy your meal, or your digestion fails to function and you do not enjoy your meal, or your cleansing mechanism fails to function and you do not release your meal . . . you would like to get your body "moving again" to improve your health and enjoyment of life's little pleasures.

The EMS and ANS, stimulated by qi, use any and all of our original release mechanisms to promote relaxation and restore our bodies to a healthy equilibrium. The body is always adjusting and fine-tuning itself. *Kiryū* releases the body's full potential to adjust and fine-tune.

And just as each person has his own anatomy and quality of qi, so each person reacts in subtly different ways to *kiryū*. There are, however, a number of characteristic responses to *kiryū*.

1. The most common, indeed universal, response is uninhibited movement. Your body may begin to twitch spasmodically, shake, shiver, or sway. You may feel you want to walk or simply lie on the floor moving your feet or legs. You may feel like flapping your arms or shaking your wrists or snapping your fingers or all of the above.

   The qi will naturally go to any part of the body that is overly tense and seek to relax it through movement. If you have bruised your right elbow, you may expect your arm to shake so that the muscles relax and the elbow joint gently moves. If you have a headache, you may expect your head to sway and your neck to swivel in order to relax the muscles along the first and second cervical vertebrae (C1 and C2). (Movements are never violent. They are always pleasurable.)

2. Yawning is a typical response. You would be surprised how many people do not yawn at all. Or cannot yawn at all. Yawning is a sign of health, a sign that the body is capable of relaxation. People who cannot yawn are destined to experience sleep

dysfunction and lower back pain. *Kiryū* stimulates the body to yawn and to stretch. When you have done *kiryū* for some months, you find that you begin to yawn and stretch just at the thought of inducing *kiryū*.

3. A release of vocalized sounds is a common response. This could be laughter or giggling, it could be a moan, it could be humming, it could be singing, or it could be noises pushed out with your breath.

4. A release of fluids frequently occurs. Tears are common in the case of women, less so in men. A woman may suddenly feel "emotional," not necessarily happy or sad, but having an irrepressible desire to cry, releasing both fluid and sounds at the same time. As the muscles in the jaw and neck relax, the body may produce a lot of saliva, which fills the mouth. Another type of fluid is mucus from the nose. Also, the body may sweat profusely without becoming feverish. The sweat may come from the entire body, or it may be localized, such as from the scalp or armpits.

5. The stomach and intestines may gurgle and rumble as they are released from their usual bondage of tension.

The effect of *kiryū* is a release from tension. You feel remarkably relaxed and clear-headed. Minor aches and pains vanish, and there is usually a sensible diminution of major aches and pains. The cumulative effect of *kiryū*—that is, to make *kiryū* a daily or thrice-weekly part of your health regimen—is to promote deep, refreshing sleep; improve digestion and muscle tone; strengthen the body's immune system; and keep the cleansing system functioning effectively.

Ultimately, the effect of qi upon the EMS and ANS will be to sensitize the organism to fulfill its potential for adaptive power.

Kiryū is the cheapest, easiest, and most effective preventive medicine measure ever devised.

Before starting the procedure for *kiryū*, a word of caution is necessary: **Because kiryū stimulates and strengthens the immune system, people with artificial body parts should not attempt the procedure. Their bodies will seek to reject the artificial "intruder."** Artificial body parts include heart valves, pins or screws in bones, breast implants, pacemakers, and artificial joints. Artificial body parts do not include dental fillings or other dental work.

I Encounter *Kiryū*

I embarked upon my *kiryū* career with great skepticism and even suspicion. Not that I thought that the process was a hoax; it seemed to me a case of mind over matter. If you believed in it enough, it would happen to you. It took me about a month to believe in my latent power and enjoy the body's natural operation of restoring itself to an optimum balance between tension and relaxation.

Our bodies are subjected to such relentless tension, both physical and psychological, that it is almost impossible to achieve total relaxation. However, as long as I do *kiryū* at least three times a week, I am never overwhelmed by tension, but *feel* calm and relaxed, and am aware that my organs are functioning healthily. Moreover, my physiology is never out of tune with the seasons. My body is guided to seasonal change as gradually and naturally as the seasons themselves.

It was Kayoko Matsuura who introduced me to *kiryū*. After she cured me of sciatica and restored my battered sciatic nerve to health, I commented, only half-jokingly, that I would have to move into her neighborhood for regular health-maintenance treatments.

"You'll never have to see me again," she said, "unless you want to because I am going to teach you a self-maintenance technique using qi to stimulate your extrapyramidal motor system and autonomic nervous system. If you stick with it, you will find it to be preventive medicine at its finest."

She was, of course, speaking Japanese, and, lacking the technical vocabulary, I had no idea what she meant by EMS or ANS. Not even finding the English equivalents proved much help. On my next visit to her, I asked for an explanation.

She put her face near mine and puffed air at me through her mouth. I blinked and quickly drew my head back.

"Your reaction was governed by the EMS," she said. "It was a reflex action. The natural unthinking movements we do all the time such as yawning and stretching and blinking and scratching and humming are all related to the EMS. Shielding your eyes or squinting from bright light is an EMS activity. Covering your ears to protect yourself from loud noises is an EMS activity. EMS is also related to the ANS and the movement and functions of organs. You can develop your EMS in the same way that you can lift weights to develop big muscles. Big muscles help you lift big things, and a well-developed EMS can bring out your full potential for health and well-being."

She did teach me the technique of *kiryū*, and my nose would probably grow if I were to write that I took to it like a duck to water. For one thing, I was very self-conscious, and the idea of my body taking control of its own movements scared me. For another thing, I mistakenly thought that Kayoko Matsuura, my savior, was the only route to salvation. She could tell me all about qi and how it had healed me, but I had strong doubts as to its efficacy without her doing whatever it was she did.

Today, I know that all *kiryū*-induced movements are natural movements. The many subtly different movements and reactions all feel good, and to be self-conscious is to introduce inhibiting tension into a healthful response. I also know that the existence of qi and its powers are greater than Kayoko Matsuura, though she may have been the foremost practitioner of her day.

Anyway, consumed by the fear of looking foolish or eccentric, I would go home, lock the doors, draw the curtains, turn off the telephone, make sure no one could possibly see me, and thus, having created a lot of unnecessary mind/body tension, was unsuccessful at stimulating the EMS. I would begin the procedure, wonder if I were doing it correctly, and then sit perfectly still for a few minutes waiting for something—I wasn't sure what—to happen. This happened every day for eight days.

On the ninth day, I went to Kayoko Matsuura's clinic and watched her instruct six women in *kiryū*. None of the women was self-conscious. In fact, they went through the procedure and enjoyed the reaction with their eyes closed. What impressed me most was how much fun, how very pleasant the exercise seemed to be to them.

They swayed and shook and made small hiccuping sounds. One woman stood up and spent a minute giving an impersonation of a child on a pogo stick. Kayoko Matsuura directed one woman to sit behind another and place her hands gently on the woman's shoulders. After about a minute, the two women were swaying in synchronized rhythm.

I stood entranced, watching. I could feel my own body yearning to move, but I was not part of the circle, and consciously restrained myself from swaying. "This is how I hold back all the time," I thought wryly, and was eager to get home and try again.

After about ten minutes, the women's movements slowly petered out until they ceased, and Kayoko Matsuura turned off the background music she had turned on when *kiryū* began. The women opened their eyes and yawned and stretched and smiled and lay quietly on the tatami flooring for a couple of minutes. Then they bowed to each other and went home.

My next attempt at *kiryū* was a success; not a stupendous success, but enough to show me that I was on the right track. After the preliminary movements to induce *kiryū*, I could feel my body quiver and then begin to shake slightly. I exhaled as deeply as I could, and my body began to move ever so slightly. Each body part—left arm, right arm, left leg, right leg, head, neck, left and right shoulder—seemed to be moving in a different direction, and yet there was an overall harmony to the movements. What appeared to be chaos was in fact well-oiled cooperation. The sensation was surprising and extremely pleasant.

I have been doing *kiryū* almost daily ever since.

After one month, I could feel how loose and relaxed my spine would become following *kiryū*. After two months, I could feel how loose and relaxed my neck and shoulders, too, would become. After three months, I realized that I could direct the flow of qi to any particular body part I wished, simply by thinking of it just prior to the onset of *kiryū*. After a year, the qi would go directly to the body part that needed it. My toes would quiver or my hands would shake or my eyelids would blink . . . whatever needed fixing, the qi would automatically go there as if targeting the problem with pinpoint precision.

If you think a year is a long time to wait for that effect, the time will pass with or without your doing *kiryū*. You might as well pass the time developing and refining your extrapyramidal motor system.

You Encounter *Kiryū*

PAIRED *KIRYŪ*

You can stimulate your EMS to launch *kiryū* by yourself or with another person. Since the latter is less complicated than the former, let us begin with that procedure.

A quiet, comfortable room is necessary. It is an aid to the flow of qi to have instrumental music playing in the background. By listening to the music with your entire body, you will not be prey to random thoughts and other workings of the mind, especially the feeling of self-consciousness. I find music with lyrics distracting. It is like having talking going on in the room, and if I know the lyrics to the song, I find myself consciously anticipating the words.

If it is possible, relax the mind/body unity by first sending qi through the spine for a minute or two. This releases tension from both giver and receiver. Having thus relaxed the giver and the receiver, proceed to the next step.

The receiver may be sitting comfortably on a backless seat or stool, or may be lying on her back. The giver will be standing or sitting behind her.

The giver first locates the receiver's Head Points Number 2 (see page 215). These are shallow grooves or trenches or depressions in the bone above the temples on both sides of the head. You will at first probably have to feel gently with your fingertips to locate the grooves (see Figure 3.1 and Figure 3.2). Most people have these grooves on their heads, and they are usually easy to locate. In cases where the grooves do not exist or can't be found, proceed with the exercise as if the grooves did exist. Certainly, the points themselves will be there.

Once the giver locates the points, he places the heart of his hands over the points. The giver and receiver should now close their eyes. The giver will begin transmitting qi into the head points. The receiver listens to the music with her body for about one minute, and then begins counting backward slowly from thirty to zero. If she reaches zero without *kiryū* inducing movement or motion, she will just continue to listen to the music and not be disappointed. The qi is flowing through her body and doing its work whether she knows it or not.

The qi will flow through her body and out of her body and into the body of the giver, "jump-starting" him into *kiryū.* The two of them will literally be sending qi back and forth to each other across the "bridge" of the giver's hands. After half a minute, the movements of the pair will become synchronized.

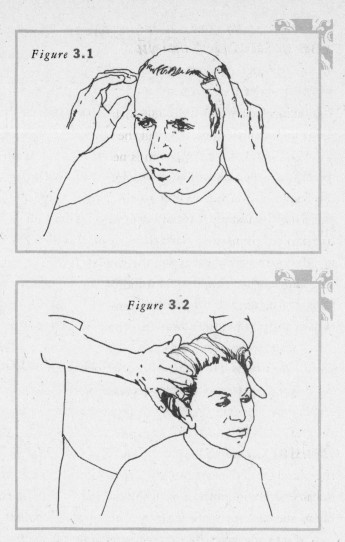

Figure **3.1**

Figure **3.2**

After three or four minutes of this, the giver will count aloud to three. At the count of three, giver and receiver will inhale together, and then compress their breaths and exhale slowly together. They open their eyes as they exhale.

If you do not wish to end *kiryū* consciously, just let the qi run its course, and all movement and motion will naturally cease. This could last as long as ten or even fifteen minutes. When that occurs, the giver will count to three, and giver and receiver will inhale together, and then compress their breaths and exhale slowly together, opening their eyes as they do so.

It may take as many as six attempts before movement is induced. If movement is not induced, do not worry, do not lose heart . . . the qi is flowing just the same.

Three fingers' width below the navel is an area called the *tanden* in Japanese. The *tanden* is considered the body's center of gravity and strength. Directly behind the *tanden* at the base of the spine is the largest nerve cluster in the body after the brain. You can always tell if *kiryū* has taken effect or if the person is "faking it," by placing your hand at the base of the spine and feeling the flow of qi. If you can feel qi moving or swirling under your palm, *kiryū* has taken effect with or without body movement.

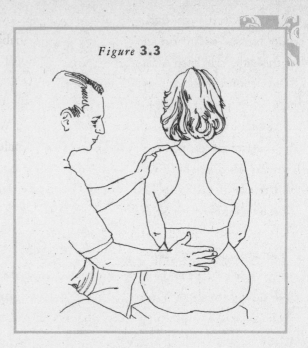

Figure **3.3**

As a result of the movement of qi, the area will be generating heat. You will be able to feel a localized warmth, usually a rhythmically pulsating warmth.

Putting qi into the base of the spine during *kiryū* is like hitting the accelerator when driving . . . it increases the flow of qi and enhances the body's response.

The giver's flow of qi will also be enhanced by keeping his hand or hands on the base of the receiver's spine (see Figure 3.3).

Solitary *Kiryū*

Choose an environment as you would to access your qi, some tranquil room or outdoor area. Put on some soothing music. Stand or sit comfortably, preferably on a backless seat of a height whereby your feet are flat on the floor.

I. Place your fingertips lightly underneath your rib cage.

1. Let your arms hang loosely at your sides. Take a deep breath through your nose, and exhale slowly through your mouth. Feel your shoulders drop and your upper body relax. Your fingers will move in about 4" and flatten your lungs, allowing for ~90% lung capacity intake instead of the usual ~55%.

Exhale until you are completely out of breath. Feel as though you have emptied your lungs and they are as flat as pancakes. Imagine that you have expelled all the old air from your lungs as if performing a cleansing operation.

Repeat this two more times, making a total of three exhalations.

2. As you inhale through your nose, try to look over your left shoulder, in order to see your own backside. Of course, you will be unable to see it. However, your chin will rise and your eyes will open wide and you will have turned and twisted your body at the waist and hips (see Figure 3.4).

   Your spine will elongate. You will feel as if you have grown half an inch to an inch, and your spine will be extremely tense. When your lungs have filled with air and your spine is at the peak of tension, exhale suddenly and powerfully through your mouth, and let your body snap back to its original position (see Figure 3.5). Your breath should come out of you in a single burst, like air from a punctured balloon.

   What you are doing is creating extreme tension along your spine, followed by instant relaxation. Now twist to the right using the same procedure. Repeat this left-right twist twice more, making a total of three times.

   This exercise on its own is an excellent way to remove tension from the neck and shoulders, and impart flexibility to the spine.

3. Place your thumbs in the palms of your hands, and squeeze them gently. Raise your hands over your head (see Figure 3.6). Close your eyes.

   Inhale deeply through your nose, and exhale powerfully through your mouth. As you exhale, squeeze your thumbs and lower your arms until your fists are at the level of your shoulders (see Figure 3.7). As your breath expires, you will feel terrific tension in your upper body and arms.

   When you run out of breath, release all the tension in your upper body. Just let yourself go limp.

   Repeat this procedure twice more, making a total of three times.

   At the final exhale, let your body go completely limp and let your hands fall to your sides or to your lap.

   Wait for *kiryū* to begin.

   It may take as many as four or five tries on consecutive days to induce movement for the first time. Once you have learned *kiryū*, the response is instantaneous.

   To end *kiryū*, take a deep breath, (compress it,) and then, as you exhale through your mouth, open your eyes slowly. *& make the uh ʌ^{uh} sound,*

This concentrates the ki in the solar plexus.

Tap your Ⓡ shoulder to totally stop it, if necessary.

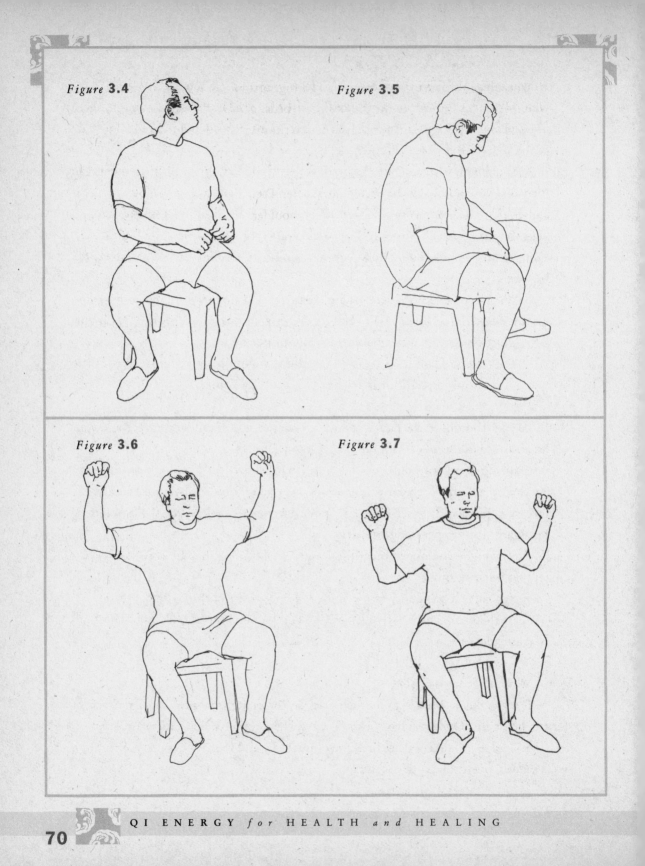

Figure 3.4

Figure 3.5

Figure 3.6

Figure 3.7

You can experience *kiryū* standing, sitting, or lying down. Many people enjoy inducing it while sitting on the side of their beds, and then lying down in bed (on their backs) once the movement has begun. On the other hand, if you have lower back-ache or leg pain, it is best to do it standing or lying on a firm surface (a bed is too soft) so that the lower limbs can move unimpeded.

Two or more people may do *kiryū* together. Each can induce his own movement, and then, touching each other on the back or shoulder, synchronized movement can be induced and a large outpouring of energy generated. I have seen as many as six people swaying in unconsciously synchronized movement (see Figure 3.8).

TRY THIS

Kiryū is an excellent means of providing a qi treatment to another person. It is strictly intuitive and requires no knowledge of treatment techniques.

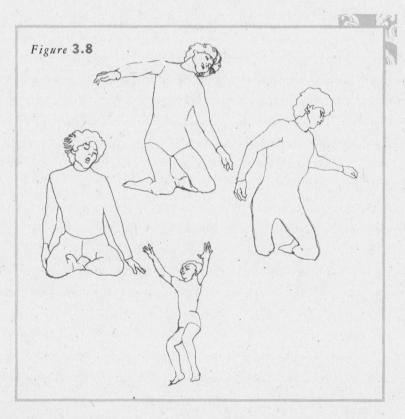

Figure **3.8**

If you have access to a massage table, this is ideal. If not, a bed is fine. The receiver should lie face-down on the table or bed. The giver should stand or sit with her left hand toward the receiver's head and her right hand toward the hips.

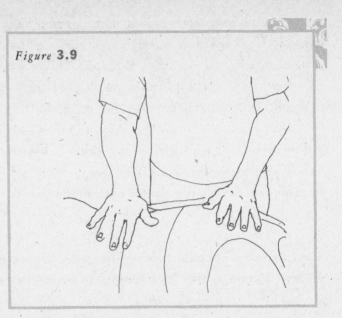

Figure **3.9**

The giver induces *kiryū* by herself. When her body responds and movement begins, she lets her hands wander all over the receiver's back.

This procedure is performed with the giver's eyes closed until the very end.

The giver's hands will naturally be attracted to any blockage of qi and will land on the spots and send qi into them until the blockage is removed (see Figure 3.9).

Her hands will then travel over the body from the head to the feet seeking to free the body from impediments to relaxation or from aches and pains. Her body will be moving as her hands busily move over the receiver's body, and this is why it is ideal to stand when performing this procedure.

The receiver is free to turn over onto his back. When the receiver is supine like this, the giver will generally find qi blockage at the solar plexus and liver. Her hands may also be drawn to the EMS grooves on either side of the head (see Figure 3.2) in order to clear away any blockage in the autonomic nervous system.

The receiver will not have a sensation of being massaged, but will feel his body being lightly brushed and stroked. It is only when blockages are found that the hands alight for any amount of time, and give qi until it is time for them to move on.

The giver ends the procedure in the usual way: ceasing her movement and feeling that her body is still, she inhales deeply through her nose, exhales, and opens her eyes slowly.

Tales of *Kiryū*

I have witnessed and heard of many interesting, even extraordinary, events of healing and health by means of *kiryū*. For example, many people who do it regularly have been saved from food poisoning by vomiting almost immediately after eating tainted food, thereby cleansing themselves before the poison has time to act. I have seen women induce *kiryū* when going into labor in order to enjoy a brief, painless childbirth. I have seen people who, feeling the onset of a migraine, induce *kiryū* and nip the migraine in the bud.

The most extraordinary case that has ever come to my attention was related to me by Richard S., a nurse in Oakland, California. Richard attended one of my qi workshops in order to receive continuing-education credits to renew his license. He had been in nursing for almost thirty years, and is, in his own words, "a hard-eyed, hard-nosed realist when it comes to medicine." In other words, he was extremely skeptical as to the existence of qi, much less its powers to heal.

On the third day of the five-day workshop, following his first attempt at *kiryū,* Richard said that he'd had an experience several months before that he wished to share with the group. The experience had been either miraculous or bizarre, depending on your interpretation, but certainly it had been inexplicable. Having learned something about qi and experienced *kiryū,* he now felt able to give a name to the phenomenon.

Richard was working in a hospital in Oakland and, through the hospital, was introduced to an elderly woman who was a quadriplegic. He became her private attendant on a part-time basis. She went to the hospital at regular intervals for tests, and Richard always accompanied her. She traveled to and from the hospital by medical transport.

One day, she was being lifted out of the transport van to be placed on a gurney for admission into the hospital when the two attendants holding her dropped her accidentally. She complained of terrible hip pain, and an X-ray was ordered. Richard saw that the hip had sustained a fracture, and the attending physician declared that at her advanced age and with her weak constitution, she would probably become enfeebled and die as a result.

Richard was beside himself with grief and frustration. He had come to love the old woman and wished deeply that there were something he could do for her. As he looked and looked at her lying in the hospital bed, he felt his hand impulsively reach out and cover her hip at the place of the fracture. His hand began to tingle, and his body began to sway slightly.

He kept his hand in place for at least thirty minutes—he had lost track of time, it was probably longer—and all the while thought healing thoughts and sent loving feelings into the old woman. He could not explain how or why, but suddenly he felt he had done enough. It was as if he had been in a dreamlike state and had returned to consciousness. He removed his hand slowly and left the old woman to sleep.

The next morning, she announced delightedly that her hip was no longer in pain, and she felt terrific. Another X-ray was ordered, and there was no sign of fracture. The attending physician, a different person from the first, studied both sets of X-rays and concluded that they were of different pelvises, because there was no way the old woman could have ever recovered from a fracture of that severity.

But Richard knew otherwise. He had been present when both sets of X-rays were taken, and had seen them together with the physicians.

He could only conclude that he had performed some sort of inexplicable miracle simply by touching her. The situation would admit no other interpretation.

There was no one he could tell this story to. For one thing, he did not understand it himself, and for another, his nurse-colleagues were just as grounded in a hard-nosed reality as he was. No one would possibly believe him, and most people would call him a crackpot.

Now, however, he could give a name and an explanation to the experience, and so was eager to tell the group.

Had anyone else but Richard told the story, I doubt that any group member, myself included, would have been convinced of its factuality. It was Richard's impressive impassivity and matter-of-factness that were so persuasive. He was a man who, had it not happened to him, would never have believed the tale. It was the happiest medical experience of his career.

The old woman was still thriving at the time he told us the story.

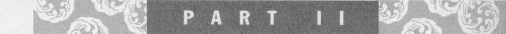

PART II

Using the Healing Power of
Qi

CHAPTER 4

The Spine and Body Systems

Some knowledge of the spinal vertebrae and head points is necessary to do the exercises in this chapter. Refer to "A Handy Guide to the Spine" and "A Handy Guide to the Head," beginning on page 212, to locate the specific vertebrae and head points.

Digestion

I look upon it, that he who does not mind his belly will hardly mind anything else.
—SAMUEL JOHNSON

The very thought makes me sick to my stomach.
—COLLOQUIAL ENGLISH EXPRESSION

The mind/body connection is nowhere more apparent than in the digestive system. Stress, worry, a failure to release negative emotions, prolonged frustration, and other emotional states can lead to a breakdown of the digestive system. You lose your appetite; nothing tastes good; what you eat does not satisfy you; you eat without even being aware you are eating, much like biting your nails; you develop acid reflux (heartburn); and finally, worst of all, you develop a polyp or polyps, or the queen of gastric problems, an ulcer or ulcers.

What is less well known is the relationship between emotional trauma and the digestive system. You can witness a horrifying sight, hear tragic news, or even imagine a tragic event and have your stomach "turn over." In extreme cases, for example, a gruesome scene of carnage or the aftermath of an unforeseen tragedy such as a terrorist attack, the sight alone can induce immediate nausea and even vomiting.

Whatever the nature of an emotional trauma—the loss of a loved one or the sight of a tragedy or a violent argument with a friend—the physical result is the same: your digestion is affected and the function of your digestive system declines. Loss of sleep usually accompanies digestive disorders.

Emotional traumas manifest themselves on the skull and the T6 vertebra.

A psychological blow produces the same trauma to the spine as a physical blow.

You can trace a line with your fingers from Head Point Number 3 to Head Point Number 5, a distance of about two and a half inches (refer to "A Handy Guide to the Head" on page 215). People who are not suffering the results of trauma will have a nice roundness between the points. People who are suffering the results of trauma will have a groove or trench or depression between the two points. Head Point Number 3 is related to gastric function and Head Point Number 5 is related to sleep. The groove between them indicates the existence of digestive and sleep problems caused by emotional trauma. The length and depth of the groove correspond to the severity of the trauma.

Within twenty-four hours of the September 11, 2001, terrorist attack, I was inundated with people complaining of gastric problems and loss of sleep. Their numbers increased rather than decreased over the next few days as the media endlessly played and replayed the horrifying sight, and it was almost impossible to go anywhere without being yet again exposed to the gruesome scene. Every person I saw had the head groove, and the groove became more pronounced the more often they witnessed the scene and their horror gave way to frustration and anger.

On a far less extreme level, a woman came in for a regular checkup. She had a plan to take her beloved father out for a special brunch on Father's Day, and was looking forward to the event. Her head was round and smooth, meaning grooveless.

On the day itself, father and daughter had a violent argument before setting off for the restaurant. Harsh words of hate were exchanged, and the woman jumped in her car and drove off alone. Before she had gone two miles, her car was rear-ended, and she became violently angry with the other driver. Again, harsh words were exchanged.

She came to see me to be treated for whiplash the day after the accident; she had a pronounced groove between Head Point Numbers 3 and 5. She had no appetite. She had awakened in the middle of the night and had been unable to return to sleep.

Emotional trauma also affects the T6 vertebra, and when a groove appears between the head points, you may be sure that T6 will not be functioning properly. Most commonly, T6 drops (sinks downward into the body). It is as if there is a gap between T5 and T7. Other times, T6 will twist to the left or right. Depending on the degree of sinking or twisting, people may feel a sharp pain in the upper back between the shoulder blades. If left unattended, the condition will lead to heartburn and even nausea.

T6 is also affected by whiplash. The vertebra tends to twist to the right or left, or even shift its position to the right or left side, depending on where one was sitting in the car when it was struck.

TREATING STOMACH DISORDERS

WEAK OR UPSET STOMACH

The Hands

Have the receiver hold out his hands, palms down. Look at the "webbing" between the thumb and forefinger. One should appear larger or more rounded than the other. Grasp this rounded point between your right thumb and forefinger, thumb on top (see Figure 4.1). Put qi in for two minutes.

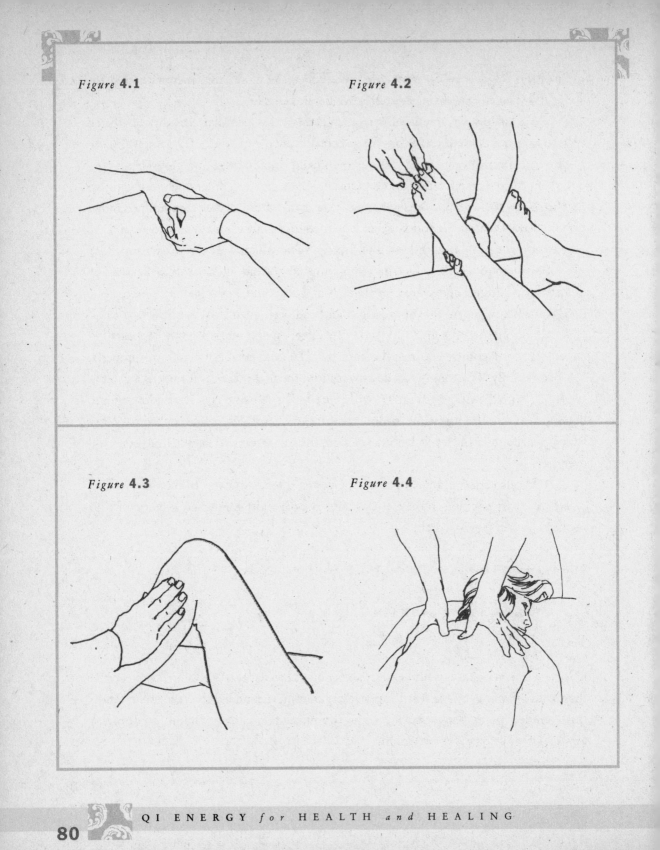

Figure **4.1**

Figure **4.2**

Figure **4.3**

Figure **4.4**

The Left Foot

The receiver lies on his back. Standing at the receiver's feet, hold the heel of the left foot with your left hand, and lift the foot slightly, about two to three inches. Grasp the tip of the second toe with your thumb and forefinger (see Figure 4.2). Your thumb should be on your left side of the receiver's toe. Put qi into the toe through your thumb. This frequently produces a response such as a growl or gurgle from the receiver's stomach. Continue for two to three minutes. Lower the foot gently and remove your hand.

The Left Leg

The receiver bends his left leg at the knee, so that the left foot is flat on the floor or table. Standing at the left side of the receiver, place your palm over the left side of the receiver's shin, and send qi from the entire palm into the shin (see Figure 4.3). Work your way slowly down the leg from the knee to the ankle, giving qi as you go.

HIATAL HERNIA

The Head

The receiver lies on her back. Standing at her left side, place the heart of your hand over Head Point Number 3, and give qi for two minutes.

The Rib Cage

You will find that one side of the rib cage is higher than the other. To determine the side, follow the procedure given on page 118. Using the procedure given on page 122 for removing tension from one side of the rib cage, lower the higher of the two sides.

DEALING WITH THE EFFECTS OF EMOTIONAL TRAUMA ON DIGESTION

Breath

Prevention is the best cure. One way to alleviate or to mitigate the traumatic effects of shock is to exhale forcefully when receiving bad news or witnessing a horrifying sight.

Most people, upon hearing tragic news, inhale suddenly and hold their breath as if frozen with horror. The entire upper body—the mind, the neck, the heart, the lungs, and the stomach—is thereby traumatized. The shock lodges in the body and is actually held inside the body until the body can cleanse itself of the shock.

In order to "close the entrance" to the body so that the shock cannot lodge within, consciously exhale powerfully and consciously feel your upper body relax the instant you receive bad news. If you are in a car and see that there is an unavoidable collision or accident just seconds away, do the same thing—exhale as powerfully as you can in order to release tension and avoid mental/physical shock by inducing flexibility into the mind/body.

Head Point Number 3

This point is located at the upper edge of the head groove produced by emotional trauma. When trauma is not present, the point is tight; however, when trauma is present, the scalp loosens at this point and it becomes soft, even spongy, usually on the right side of the point.

The receiver should be on her stomach. The giver stands to her right and places the heart of his right hand on Head Point Number 3. Give qi for three minutes or until you feel the scalp begin to firm up.

T6 Vertebra

The giver now stands at the receiver's head and places his thumbs alongside T6. Pressing down gently but firmly with the thumbs, extend both hands horizontally along the receiver's back and send qi into the back with both hands, thumbs included (see Figure 4.4).

The giver should be aware of the rise and fall of the receiver's back as she inhales and exhales. After one minute, exhale together with the receiver, pressing down with your thumbs as you do so, as if to help expel all the air in her lungs. When your breath terminates, release your grip, and remove your hands gently.

This procedure is beneficial for those suffering from heartburn.

The Liver

The liver is located directly below the rib cage on the right side. To locate it, place your right hand on the rib cage and slide it down until the left side of your hand is no longer on the rib cage but directly below it and touching the last rib. Your hand is now over the liver (see Figure 4.5).

Lower Abdomen

The receiver is still on her back. Locate her navel. Measure three fingers' width from the bottom of the navel, and place your right middle finger on that point. Cover the finger with your left middle finger, and, pressing gently but firmly, put qi into the spot for one minute (see Figure 4.6).

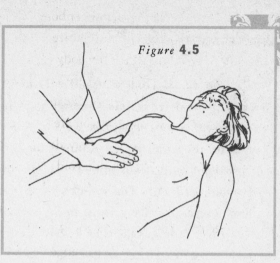

*Figure **4.5***

Head Groove

The receiver turns over onto her stomach. The giver feels for the head groove. It should not be as pronounced as it was. Cover the groove with your right hand, and send qi directly into it for two minutes.

Repeat this procedure daily for five days, and the head groove will disappear together with major digestion problems.

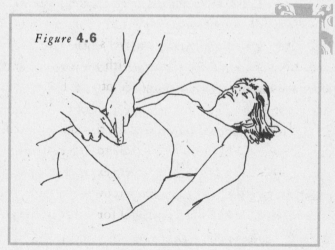

*Figure **4.6***

Ron was sixty-one years old and had very poor digestion accompanied by acid reflux. He almost always had heartburn after meals and moved his bowels only twice a week. What was notable in Ron's case was that he also suffered from scoliosis, or curvature of the spine. His spine bowed out to the right from T5 to L2, a total of ten vertebrae, creating a pronounced hump. The scoliosis caused him a number of other discomforts, in fact, too many to list in this section on digestion.

Not only was his spine curved to the right, but his T6, T10, T11, and T12 were twisted to the right.

I relaxed Ron's spine, and then gave qi to each vertebra, followed by qi alongside the four twisted vertebrae. After four treatments, T5, T6, T12, L1, and L2 "returned to the fold," meaning that they straightened out of the curve and into alignment. At the same time, T6 and T12 were untwisted, and my qi now flowed into them and along their neural pathways with ease.

Ron's acid reflux disappeared, and his bowel movements grew more frequent. It took three more treatments before he was moving his bowels daily. It took nine treatments to relieve him of all his discomforts, and a total of twenty-four treatments to restore his entire spine to alignment and his hump to disappear.

Looking at Ron today, you would never know that he suffered from scoliosis for forty-six years.

CASE HISTORY

Laura was an eighty-year-old woman who had lived a hard, tragedy-filled life. Her husband, who had shared her life since they were teenagers, was her sole source of happiness and fulfillment. To make him a special birthday dinner each year was her enduring delight. She saved what she could from her limited housekeeping money week by week in order to prepare him an extravagant meal.

On the morning of his eighty-second birthday, she awoke to find that her husband, beside her in bed, had died in his sleep during the night. His death had been quiet and painless. Laura was, of course, grief-stricken.

She was given antidepressants and sleeping pills to help her get through the month following her husband's death. She came to see me three months following his death, complaining of an acrid taste in her mouth that never left her. Nothing tasted good, no food appealed to her, her chest felt tight, and her heart felt as if it were being squeezed. Her only grandchild was being married in four weeks, and she wanted to be able to enjoy the wedding reception.

I immediately looked for a head groove, and found a long and deep one. The right side of her Head Point Number 3 was spongy, almost squishy, her rib cage had contracted on both sides, and her stomach and organs had risen. Her heart really was being squeezed. Her T6 was nowhere to be found. It was as if it had walked off the job.

I restored the T6 to its rightful position and invigorated it with qi. I lowered her organs by lowering her rib cage and stimulated her liver to cleanse her. I spent about five minutes putting qi into the groove itself.

The bitter sensation in her mouth diminished with each treatment, but it took six treatments before the head groove disappeared completely and Laura's sense of taste returned fully. She thoroughly enjoyed the wedding reception.

Body Cleansing

The most fastidious feline must stand in awe of the compulsive cleansing mechanism of the human body. Every breath, every heartbeat, every blink, every sneeze, every "you name it," all are part of the great cleansing process. Everything we put into our bodies, whether it be air, food, aspirin, or water, has to be removed from it in a transmuted form.

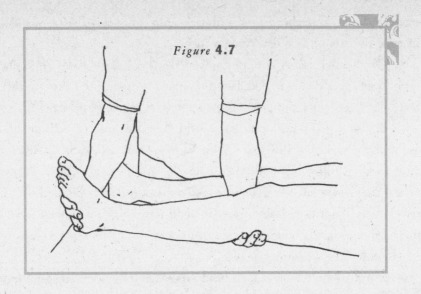

Figure **4.7**

The most obvious cleansing mechanisms are the urinary tract and the gastrointestinal (GI) tract. You can also cleanse through your mouth by vomiting or coughing up phlegm. You cleanse through your lungs with each breath. You can cleanse through your nose by sneezing or secreting mucus. You can cleanse through your eyes with tears and mucus. You can cleanse through your ears with wax. You can cleanse through your skin with sweat. You can cleanse through your mind with sleep and dreams and sorrow and laughter. Women cleanse through their reproductive system by means of flexibility of the pelvis.

THE URINARY TRACT

The urinary tract is the most sensitive system in the body to fatigue and exhaustion. For example, when the lungs need strengthening and invigorating due to smoking or illness, the urinary tract will also lose its vigor as the body works hard to cope with the poor cleansing performance of the lungs. The same holds true when liver function declines.

The performance of the urinary tract is directly related to the integrity of L3, but is also related to the kidneys, which are controlled by T11.

When the urinary tract tires or is unable to function to capacity, the inside of the left thigh tightens, becomes a blotchy red, and is tender to the touch. In some people,

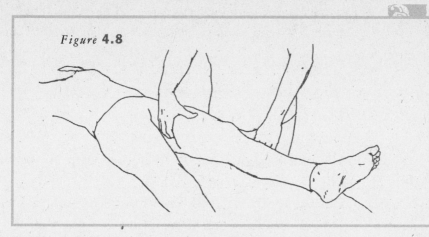

Figure **4.8**

it is the inside of the right thigh that presents these symptoms, but in my experience, about 80 percent of urinary problems are manifested on the left inner thigh.

To treat this problem you may follow this procedure:

1. The receiver lies on his back. The giver stands on the receiver's right near his feet. Place your right hand on the sole of the receiver's left foot. With your right hand in the center of the arch, place your left hand under the left knee so that the back of the knee is resting on the palm of your hand. Pressing firmly with your right hand, send qi to your left hand for one minute (see Figure 4.7).

2. With the receiver still on his back, he opens his legs about eight inches. The giver is at his left. The giver places the fingers of his right hand under the left thigh where it joins the crotch. There will be a "tight" line. Bend your fingers and squeeze as if scooping, sending qi as you do (see Figure 4.8). This will loosen the entire line.

3. The most tender spot along the line is usually close to the knee. Find it and give it direct qi with the heart of the hand for one minute.

4. The receiver turns over onto his stomach. The kidneys are located just beneath where the ribs end, at T12. Standing at the receiver's left, the giver places a hand over each kidney and sends qi from the whole hand for one minute.

Finally, when the urinary tract is performing poorly, it is good to drink a lot of fluids, especially water. In cold months, warm water is particularly good for stimulating urinary tract function.

CASE HISTORY

My bout with sciatica lasted two years. During that time, it never occurred to me that I was not urinating easily because of the local sciatic pain that arose whenever I squeezed my bladder in order to urinate. It also never occurred to me that my failure to completely relieve myself of urine meant that toxins were remaining in my body. In fact, my skin was blotchy, and I later realized that it was from the toxins, for within a week of the toxins being released through urine, my skin returned to its pristine unblotchy self.

While Kayoko Matsuura was working on me, she felt the inside of my right thigh and remarked, "You haven't had a good pee in months. It doesn't gush out like it should." The local area was indeed extremely sensitive, even painful. She proceeded to treat me in the manner described above. I am one of the few people whose urinary tract resonates on the right leg. Anyway, when her treatment was complete, the inside of the thigh was no longer tender.

I was able to urinate easily and painlessly thereafter. My skin cleared up and my right inner thigh never pained me again.

THE INTESTINES

The function of the intestines is related to L2. When L2 is tight and without resilience, the digestive system and elimination are slow and dull, and there is a tendency to constipation.

Antibiotics are cleansed from the body through the intestines, and it is helpful to maintain good intestinal function when on a course of antibiotics by drinking a lot of ionized water or water containing electrolytes. Ionized water is also very helpful for alleviating the side effects of anesthesia.

A person who feels discomfort or even pain in L2 will be eliminating poorly. The discomfort indicates that the vertebra is out of alignment. Realigning the vertebra will produce diarrhea, which is a cleansing activity.

To treat constipation and invigorate intestinal function:

1. With the receiver on her stomach, the giver stands at her left. L4 is at the top of the pelvis, and L2 is about two to two and a half inches above it. When you have located it, place your thumbs in the groove on either side of the vertebra and, pressing gently but firmly, put qi into the points for a minute (see Figure 4.9).

    To end, synchronize your breath with the receiver's, and on your final exhale, release your thumbs quickly when you have run out of breath.

2. Place your right hand on the back of the receiver's right knee (see Figure 4.10). Send qi into the spot through the heart of your hand. Do this for three minutes.

3. The receiver turns over onto her back. The giver is at the receiver's right. Place your right hand on the abdomen so that the heel of your thumb is on the navel, and the rest of your hand is below and to the left of the navel (see Figure 4.11). Put qi into this spot for two minutes, and withdraw your hand slowly.

A blow or blows to the head and upper body frequently lead to vomiting and diarrhea. The above treatment will speed up this natural cleansing process and realign L2.

THE LIVER

More and more, I respect the role of the liver in the body, and suspect that its function is even more profound than we know. Reading the liver to know if it is active or passive, sensitive or insensitive, is part of every qi treatment. A "plumped-up" liver with qi flowing steadily through it is a sign that the treatment has been a success.

To improve liver function and invigorate the liver:

Figure **4.9**

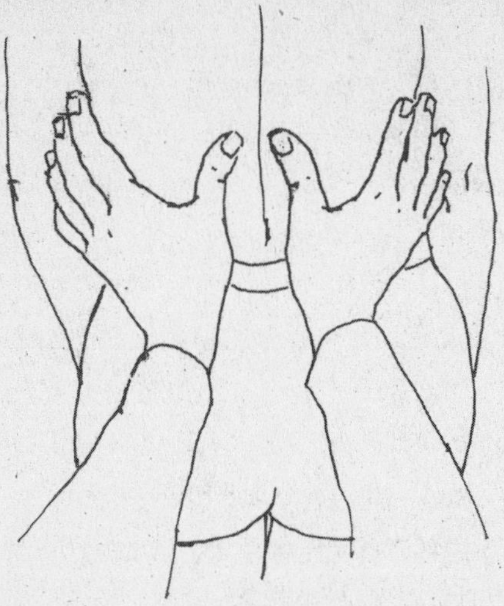

Figure **4.10**

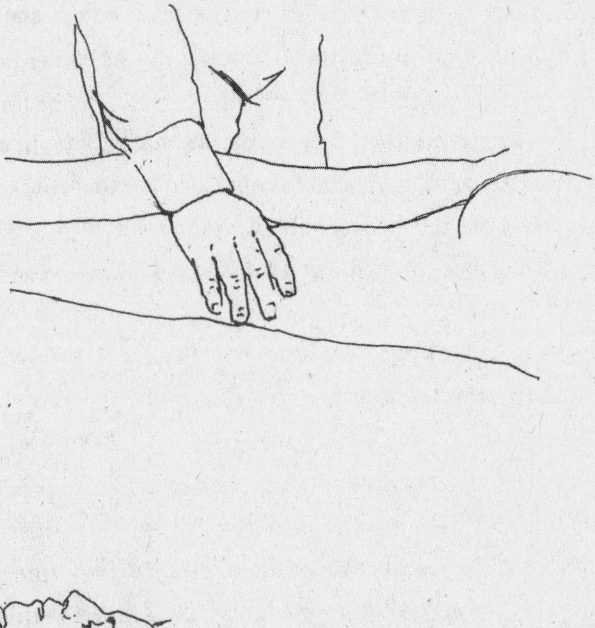

Figure **4.11**

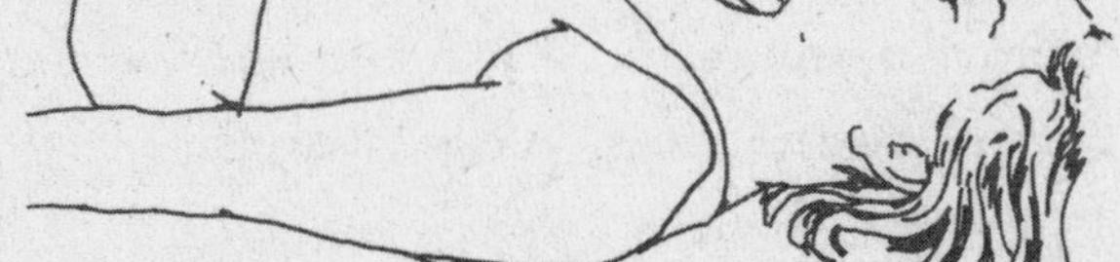

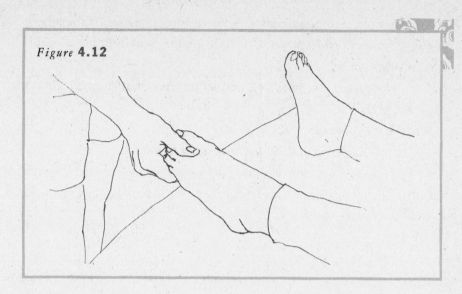

Figure **4.12**

1. The receiver lies on his back, legs outstretched. The giver goes to the left foot. Grasping the first two toes firmly, the giver pulls the foot outward and toward the floor so that it forms a flat plane. The point for qi is at the bottom of the second toe between it and the third toe. Place your right thumb over this point, and send qi in for two minutes (see Figure 4.12). Withdraw your fingers slowly when you are done.

2. Send direct qi to the liver for two minutes as explained on page 122.

CASE HISTORY

Judy, a middle-aged woman with no particular health issues, came in complaining of feeling listless and just not as perky as usual. Further, she had a tightness just below her rib cage on the right, and when she put her hand there, she could feel the spot emitting warmth.

I felt her liver. It was small, tight, and sluggish. The qi did not flow in smoothly, and the liver did not respond to direct, local qi. I worked on the point between her toes for a couple of minutes, and then went back to giving direct qi. After three minutes, her liver suddenly "exploded." That is the only word I can use to describe the feeling. It was as if it had been instantly transformed from a ninety-eight-pound weakling into a world-class muscle man.

The response was so strong and so unexpected that Judy almost leapt off the table.

"What happened? What was that?" she cried.

"It was your liver waking up from hibernation," I replied.

She felt that her entire abdominal cavity was filled with healthy warmth. She phoned a few days later to say that her energy had returned and she was feeling great.

THE SKIN

The skin is the largest and most visible organ of the body. We cleanse through the skin, and we regulate body heat through the skin. People who do not sweat are, first of all, odd, and second, tend to suffer from mild acne or blotchy skin.

The skin is related to the function of the brain and nervous system, which is why it turns red when we are embarrassed, or livid when we are frightened. The skin is very susceptible to psychological factors, particularly those deriving from emotional stress. It is not uncommon for people of any age to break out in pimples or rashes when prolonged emotional stress results in tension in the neck and head.

L1 is the vertebra responsible for cleansing the brain and nervous system, and it is to that vertebra we must first turn when dealing with skin problems. The method is the same as that for aligning and imparting flexibility to the other vertebrae: place your thumbs on either side of the vertebra, and give qi for one to two minutes.

Skin problems are frequently related to sugar intake, meaning the more sugar we eat, the more skin problems we have. Liquor, especially wine and hard liquor, is rich in sugar. For people with skin problems, particularly psoriasis, liquor should be avoided or taken in moderation.

The mind and body should be relaxed, and to that end, the person can do *kiryū* daily or even twice daily. It is also good for a second person to send qi into the entire spine in order to restore flexibility to L1 in the context of collaborating with its vertebral colleagues.

Night sweats are both a cleansing function and a natural auto-alignment function. Night sweats occur when the body relaxes and adjusts itself spontaneously. They usually occur twice during the night—within the first hour of sleep, and again in the early morning. Night sweats are a clear sign of local cleansing and adjusting. They do not indicate a full-body change, but a local and specific change, though where this change takes place is not always evident. Night sweats occur at a time of infection, indicating that the body is both fighting the specific infection and adjusting to cope with it. People with sensitive bodies, such as people who do *kiryū* on a regular basis, will experience night sweats throughout the year as their bodies cope with external stimuli that are not always beneficial.

MENSTRUATION

A female is born with her full complement of eggs. It is only a matter of time until she becomes fertile, in other words, capable of putting a viable egg in a location where it is likely to encounter a sperm. Should that encounter not occur, the egg is cleansed from the body through menstruation, and a fresh, new egg is sent out to wait again.

Menstruation is one of the most important cleansing mechanisms in a woman's body, and is very susceptible to changes, both physical and emotional, in the woman's life. For example, chemotherapy following cancer can cause a cessation of periods, as can stress at the workplace.

It is the ovaries that launch the egg into position, a process called ovulation. It is the ovaries that stimulate the pelvis to open at the time of menses, and close following the end of menses, just like in the case of childbirth. In a healthy woman, there are two ovaries, but only one works each month. The ovaries work in alternation, right-left-right-left, so that an equilibrium of tension and relaxation is achieved. Neither ovary is overworked, and so each can fulfill its function dutifully and effectively.

Many women, in fact I should say most women, do not feel themselves ovulating and do not know which ovary is at work at any given month. There are two ways of ascertaining which ovary is functioning, and once you have done that, it is easy to keep track of the alternation between left and right.

The first way is through soreness or tenderness in a breast. One breast will usually be more tender to the touch before the onset of menses. The tender breast corresponds to the working ovary. If the right breast is sore, then the right ovary is functioning that month and the left is at rest. Should there be no tenderness, the

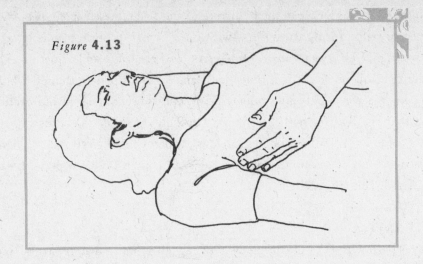

Figure **4.13**

woman should lie on her back, hands at her sides. Using the index, middle, and ring fingers of the opposite hand, she should feel along the side of her breast where it meets the rib cage. There is likely to be a tender spot on one of the breasts.

This tender spot is also easy to locate by means of qi, for it will usually be warmer than the surrounding area.

The giver can quickly locate the tender spot by cupping the hand, placing the palm slightly above the base of the breast, and moving the hand slowly over the area. The tender point will send heat into the heart of the hand (see Figure 4.13).

Once located, put qi into that spot until it ceases to be tender. Usually, the middle finger, the longest, is the easiest to use. Putting qi into the tender point of each breast each month should be done about one week before menses is due to begin.

The other way to locate the working ovary is by sight or by touch. This can be done only between the time of ovulation and the beginning of menses, a time frame of roughly two weeks.

The ovaries are usually located about three inches above the pubic bone and to the sides. In most women, the ovaries are visible when she lies naked on her back. There appear to be two very slight mounds that may be seen from the side, in silhouette as it were. One of the mounds will be quivering slightly, the other will be inert. The quivering side is the working ovary. If you place your hands on the two spots, they will feel similar to marshmallows, pleasantly soft.

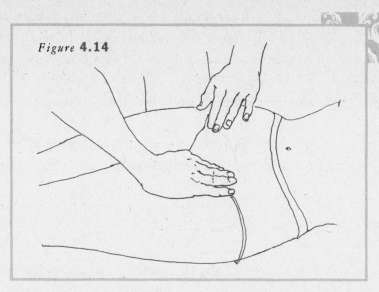

Figure **4.14**

Again, it is possible to locate the ovaries using qi. The woman, lying on her back, can find her ovaries by touch, and direct the giver to them. He places the index, middle, and ring fingers of his left hand on her right ovary, and his right hand on her left ovary (see Figure 4.14). Sending qi into both ovaries, he awaits a response. One will respond by becoming warm, while the other will not change at all, but feel cold and dull. This unresponsive ovary is the resting ovary.

For women who have irregular periods, or severe cramping, or PMS

The first thing to do is to locate a working ovary, as this will be the point of departure for your monthly regimen.

The day after the menstrual blood changes color from red to brown (usually the fourth or fifth day of the period), qi should be put into the resting ovary. If the right ovary worked for that cycle, then put qi into the left ovary for three consecutive days. Each day will take less time as the working ovary slows down and the resting ovary becomes active. There is no stipulated amount of time for giving qi. It varies according to the sensitivity of the individual. Just keep sending qi until you feel the silent ovary begin to quiver. The receiver should feel the ovary swing into action.

A woman can do her own ovarian procedure. She lies on her back and sends qi through the resting ovary with her breath. She inhales through her nose, and exhaling, she imagines a white vapor leaving her resting ovary and ascending to the ceiling. Then she takes another inhalation through the nose and exhalation through the ovary, keeping up a rhythmic breathing pattern. She should place her hands over, but not touch, the ovaries in order to ascertain that qi is passing through the resting one.

With each passing month, her confidence will grow and her ovaries will respond more strongly to the qi, which may be felt as high as eight to ten inches above the ovary.

CASE HISTORY

Elinor had a child when she was twenty-five years old, but though she and her husband tried conscientiously to have another, she did not get pregnant.

She came to see me at the age of thirty-six. We went through three menstrual cycles together, and I was able to ascertain that only her right ovary was functioning. Her left never functioned, so the right was sorely overworked. In fact, every other month, her right ovary pained her as though it was cramping up. Her cycles were as regular as clockwork, but without a functioning second ovary, she had slight chance of conceiving. She also suffered from mild lower backache, centered on L3 and L4.

It took three more cycles, but with regular application of qi to the left ovary, and with qi stimulation to L3 and L4, she conceived in the seventh cycle after commencing treatment.

L3 regulates the movement of the pelvis. Without the left ovary stimulating it, her pelvis barely moved each month, which is also an impediment to pregnancy. It takes a nice, fully closed pelvis to get pregnant. This is why nursing mothers usually do not get pregnant (though I have known several exceptions to this rule), as stimulating the breasts keeps the pelvis open. It was necessary to restore the flexibility of L3 to ensure that both sides of the pelvis opened and closed harmoniously.

L4 is related to the reproductive system, especially the cleansing of the system. By restoring flexibility to this vertebra, the body was inclined to gear up to get pregnant.

Elinor had a baby girl. Thanks to the newfound flexibility of her pelvis, the birth was brief and uneventful.

Muscles and Bones

Upper and lower back pain, stiff shoulders, sore neck, stiff arms, TMJ, and other aches and pains all derive from the same source: a loss of flexibility. Whether this loss is induced by a blow, by a twisted vertebra, or by constant and chronic stress, the result is the same.

The application of qi provides a quick and effective remedy to these aches and pains. By "quick and effective remedy," I do not mean that following a single twenty-minute treatment the sufferer leaps up off the massage table and whirls like Fred Astaire. I mean that after five or six treatments, the person will realize that the pain is greatly diminished and the range of motion is enlarged.

Bones do not move of their own accord. Dancing skeletons are the products of special-effects teams and have nothing to do with Nature's handiwork. It is muscles and tendons and ligaments that move our bones. However, these body parts do not move of their own accord. They must be given commands.

There are several types of nerve receptors, called spindles, that have their home in the muscles, tendons, and ligaments. These spindles are, or try to be, in constant communication with General Headquarters (the brain) in order to carry out orders instantly. It is through their efforts that you can play the clarinet, kick a ball, or pick your nose (perhaps the most common unconscious behavior of the human race).

Unfortunately, the channels linking the spindles to the nervous system are not always open and clear. A physical or psychological blow will impair communication between spindle and nervous system. So, too, will prolonged stress. Spindles cry out to the nervous system for guidance and leadership, but no response is forthcoming. Spindles are soon no longer able to fulfill their original function of stimulating muscles to move as smoothly and effectively as they might. The muscle or tendon then loses its flexibility, and the upshot is ache or, in a chronic situation, pain.

Muscles do not want to be stiff. Bones do not want to be out of alignment. And nobody wants to be in pain. Qi acts directly on the afflicted spindles and induces them to relax the stiff muscle(s) by providing them with the commands they have been asking for. The muscles have been seeking health, or at least a respite from ongoing discomfort. Qi provides them the opportunity. Once the muscle(s) relaxes, channels of communication reopen, and aches and pains disappear.

"Anatomy is destiny," wrote Freud, and that includes the psychological part of our anatomy. Our psychological problems always find a home in our bodies, the body part varying according to the individual. The physical manifestation of our problems is tension.

All of us have feelings of anger, indignation, hostility, frustration, and more at one time or another. These feelings either alone or in combination produce tension. Then we have worries—money, our children's louche best friends, the yenta gabbing on her cell phone in a colossal SUV—which add to our store of tension. On top of it all, we have deadlines to meet, unpleasant customers to deal with, nagging responsibilities, and caretaking our elderly family members. When you think about it, it is amazing just how resilient we are; one would think we would be paralyzed by all the tension in our lives.

And in fact, to some extent we are paralyzed in our muscles and bones, and so we seek relief.

As a rule, men and women carry their tension in different places.

Women often carry tension in one of the shoulders around the shoulder blade. The tense shoulder usually corresponds to the side on which she wears her handbag. Upper back tension is exacerbated by wearing high heels. Women also often carry tension in their buttocks. They are unaware that they are clenching their buttocks from the moment they stand up until the moment they sit down. One side will be tighter than the other and will correspond to the tense shoulder. Prolonged tension in the buttocks causes the sacrum to twist and dig into the surrounding muscle. The resulting pain is stupendous, and frequently runs down the leg. It is like being cut by a knife. This pain is usually misdiagnosed as sciatica.

Men, on the other hand, tend to clench their jaws when they are tense. As a result, Head Points Number 4 become so tight that they fill out the "dimple" that is normally there. When this area becomes tense, the function of the salivary glands is impaired, and dry mouth ensues. This is not bad in and of itself, but as digestion begins in the mouth, the absence of saliva results in digestive problems.

Policemen and professional athletes chew gum in order to make saliva, as the occupational tension in their lives has them clenching their jaws. I have a married couple as patients who are both police officers. They have to chew gum in order to kiss, their mouths are so dry. Their lips are normally like sandpaper. Both suffer from indigestion.

Chronic tension in the Head Points Number 4 also leads to tinnitis and/or loss of hearing. The neck becomes extremely tense, and the muscles running along the side of the neck become like steel cables. Range of motion is inhibited, and in extreme cases, a person cannot turn his head easily enough to use the side mirrors when driving.

TREATMENTS FOR MUSCLE ACHES AND PAINS

NECK ACHE

Head Points Number 4

The receiver is seated, and the giver is seated or standing behind him. Place your middle fingers on Head Points Number 4, and press firmly but gently. Send qi into the points for two minutes. As the muscles relax, your fingers will go deeper into the points.

C2 Point

The receiver is seated, and the giver is seated behind him. Just at the base of the skull where it curves into the neck is a slight hollow or depression. Run your thumb over the hard bone of the skull, and where it slides into the soft neck, that is the hollow (see Figure 4.15). Both your left and right thumbs should be able to locate the points without difficulty.

Place your other fingers on

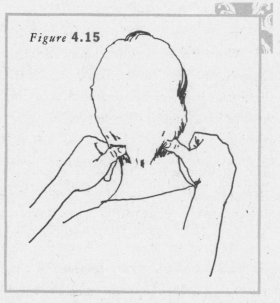

Figure **4.15**

the sides of the receiver's head. Having done this, tell the receiver to open his eyes, roll his eyeballs upward, and keep them in that position. Pull the receiver's head back so that the chin goes up. Your thumbs should sink into the C2 points at the base of the skull (see Figure 4.16). Keeping firm pressure with your thumbs, send qi with all of your fingers. The receiver's spine will tense. Maintaining this tension, continue sending qi for a minute.

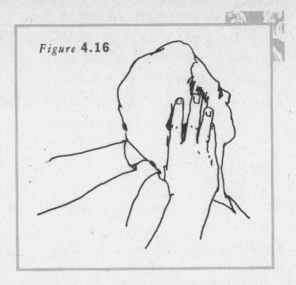

Figure **4.16**

At the end of the minute, release the pressure of your thumbs suddenly and restore the head to its normal position, chin down. In this posture, continue sending qi with your fingers for another minute, and then withdraw your hands slowly as you exhale.

Solar Plexus

The receiver lies on his back. The giver is seated or standing at the receiver's right. Place the left hand under the receiver's neck, so that your index, middle, and ring fingers are cradling the neck. Turn the neck slowly to the left and right. One direction will feel more comfortable than the other. Place the heart of your right hand over the solar plexus, located just beneath the center of the rib cage. Holding the neck in the more comfortable direction, send qi into the solar plexus and neck for three minutes (see Figure 4.17). Remove your hands slowly.

Base of Neck

The receiver is still on his back. The giver sits behind him. Place your thumbs on the spots where the neck meets the shoulders. There will be a "dimple" at these points. Pressing firmly but gently with your thumbs, send qi into these points for one minute. Release your thumbs suddenly when you are through.

STIFF SHOULDERS AND ARMS

First, perform the procedure given on page 49 ("A Hello to Arms").

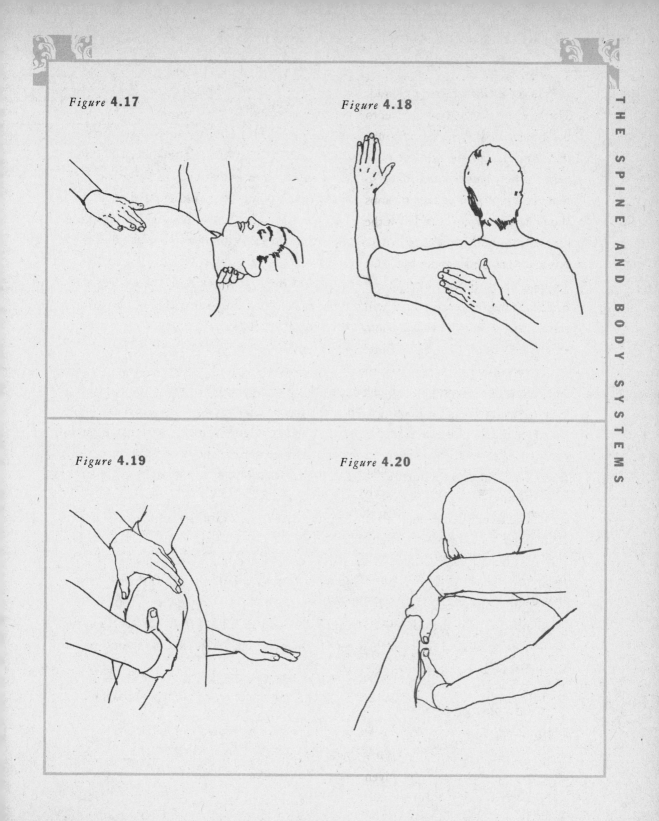

Figure **4.17**

Figure **4.18**

Figure **4.19**

Figure **4.20**

Shoulder Blades

The receiver is seated, and the giver is seated or standing behind him. The receiver bends the elbow of the side with the stiff shoulder to form a right angle, fingers pointing upward. (For the purpose of illustration, we will use the left shoulder.) The receiver slowly raises his arm over his head. At some point, he will feel that the movement is stiff or is causing discomfort. At this point, he should tense his arm and shoulder. The giver places her whole hand over the tight, "stuck" area, and sends qi in for two minutes. If the location is vague rather than precise, place your hand on the upper part of the shoulder blade (see Figure 4.18).

To end this procedure, the giver counts to three, at which signal both giver and receiver exhale forcefully. At the end of the exhalation, the giver withdraws her hand slowly, while the receiver lets his arm drop loosely to his side.

Shoulder

The receiver sits comfortably, preferably with his eyes closed. The giver sits perpendicular to the receiver's stiff shoulder. The giver locates a point two to three inches below the top of the shoulder, in the center of the rounded bulge of muscle. Placing one hand on top of the shoulder to steady it, put the thumb over the shoulder point and press firmly but gently (see Figure 4.19). Send qi for two minutes, and release the pressure of your thumb quickly to terminate the procedure.

The receiver continues to sit. The giver sits behind him. To work on the right shoulder, the giver places his right hand under the receiver's armpit so that the right thumb is on the back of the receiver's shoulder and the rest of the hand lies on the chest. Place your left hand over the collarbone (clavicle) so that your left thumb meets your right thumb (see Figure 4.20). The thumbs will form a single, vertical line along the joint where the shoulder is attached to the body. Pressing firmly but gently with both thumbs, send qi into the shoulder for three minutes. Release your thumb pressure quickly to terminate the procedure.

LOWER BACK PAIN

Most lower backache, perhaps as much as 80 percent, is related to L1, L3, or L5.

L 1

Typically, the ache or pain around L1 does not become severe enough to impede movement. Sufferers can still function adequately. L1 rarely, if ever, protrudes or sinks. It usually moves to the right or left, or up or down.

The first lumbar vertebra is related to the cleansing of the brain and nervous system, and thus is also related to the neck. An abnormality in L1 frequently translates itself into skin problems, including acne, eczema, and psoriasis. There are often psychological factors at work that impede the efficient operation of L1, which in turn impedes the skin's ability to cleanse. When the excretory/cleansing function of the skin is impaired, psychological stress and physical tension remaining in the head and neck can literally pollute the body by allowing a buildup of toxins that would normally be expelled by the skin.

When L1 loses its flexibility, besides backache and skin problems, one's mental alertness and physical sensitivity decline. If left untreated over time, this can lead to a loss of all appetites, including sexual appetite. People become quite immersed in their own thoughts, most of which are pointless or anxiety-producing, and lose interest in the physical and sensory world.

When there is discomfort in L1, the first thing to do is the procedure for alleviating neck ache, proceeding from there to the shoulders. After adjusting those parts, put a lot of qi into the Achilles tendons and ankles. Then move to the vertebra itself, and put direct qi into it.

L 3

People with pain in L3 suffer the most severe lower back pain, especially when L3 is twisted. One feels unable to walk due to pain. The activities of daily life are impeded. A twist in L3 can produce sciatica in one or both legs.

To treat L3 pain, the receiver lies on his back, legs stretched out below him so that the inner ankles are almost touching. The pain will probably be greater on one side of the spine than the other. If there is sciatica, one leg will be more affected than the other. The giver goes to the receiver's feet and takes the more painful leg by the heel, and gently opens it twelve inches. In other words, there will now be a space of twelve inches between the inner ankles (see Figure 4.21).

Raise the leg and bend the knee so that the sole of the foot is flat on the floor

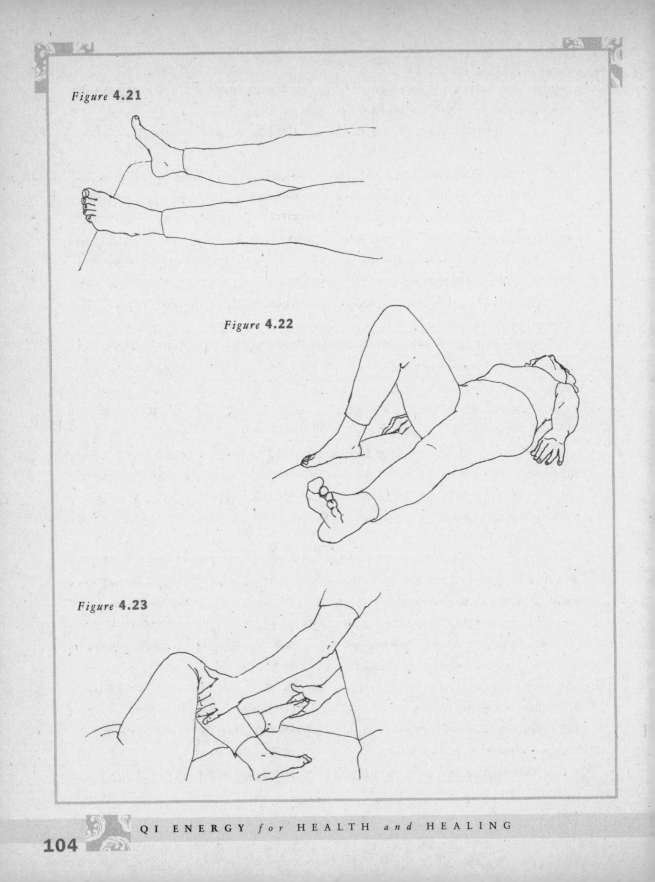

Figure **4.21**

Figure **4.22**

Figure **4.23**

or table, the heel of the foot being as close to the receiver's body as possible (see Figure 4.22).

The giver places her thumb just below the knee and to the side of the shin. There will be a dimple, perhaps tender, for the thumb to rest in. With her other hand, the receiver takes the toes of the opposite foot, and turns them to herself, holding them down almost flat against the floor or table. Now, putting qi into her thumb, she presses into the side of the shin so that the receiver's leg is pushed about five inches toward himself (see Figure 4.23). The receiver will feel a rush of tension to his L3.

The giver holds this position, toes and knee pointing toward each other, for thirty seconds, and then quickly releases her hands. The foot and leg will spring back to their original positions. Repeat this one more time, and then slowly lower the raised leg back to the table.

The receiver now turns over onto his stomach. The giver puts direct qi into L3 for two minutes.

L5

A loss of flexibility to L5 impairs back-and-forth movements. For example, it is painful first thing in the morning to bend over the sink to wash your face. Side-to-side movements do not produce pain, but bending from the waist is always painful. Treat L5 discomfort the way you would sacral pain, described below.

SACRAL PAIN

The sacrum, like the other bones in the spine, moves quite a bit, and frequently twists or tilts. When this occurs and remains in a fixed position, a shooting pain, often mistaken for sciatica emanating from the lumbar vertebrae, travels down the leg.

The receiver lies facedown. One of the buttocks will be out of alignment, meaning one side will be "plump" and high, while the other will be "flat" and low. The "flat" and low buttock is out of alignment. To check this, place the edge of your hands at the lower edge of the buttocks (see Figure 4.24). Stand on the side of the receiver opposite to the "flat" and low buttock. Curving your right hand, place it under the fleshy part of the hip, and pull upward and toward yourself so that the buttock "plumps up." Cover your right hand with your left hand, and send qi into the spot with your entire hand for two minutes (see Figure 4.25). Release your hands quickly on an exhalation.

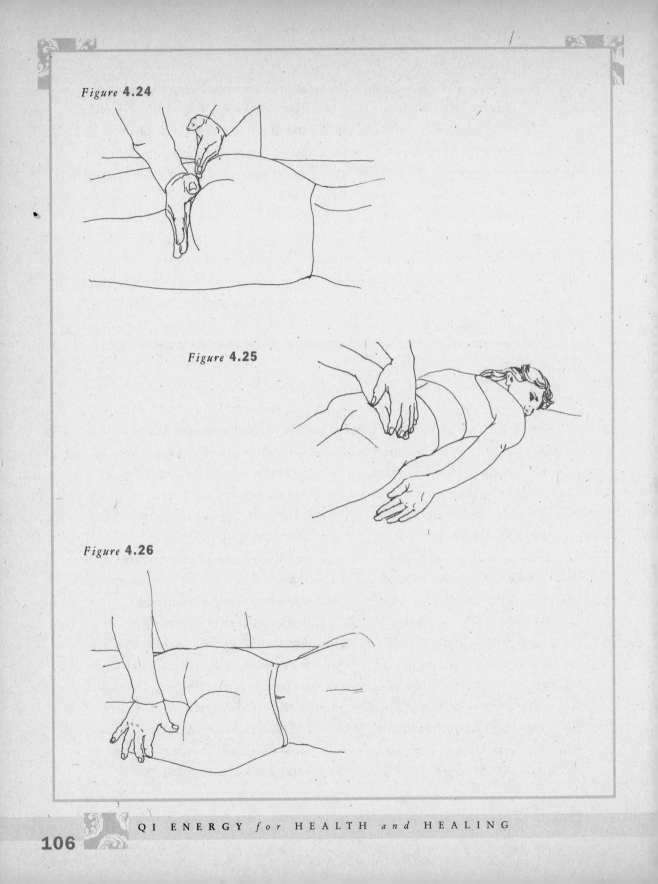

Figure **4.24**

Figure **4.25**

Figure **4.26**

Check the measurement of the buttocks again. They should be even. If they are not, place your right thumb in the center of the back of the upper thigh just beneath the unaligned buttock. Pressing down firmly, send qi into the spot for thirty seconds (see Figure 4.26). Release quickly, move your thumb down an inch, and send qi into the spot for thirty seconds. Repeat this procedure until you have gone from the lower edge of the buttock to the top of the back of the knee.

CASE HISTORY

Denise was a forty-six-year-old nurse working in a large hospital. Her work was physically demanding. It involved lifting heavy objects (including patients) and bending and twisting from the waist and hips in tight spaces.

She began experiencing short bursts of shooting pain in her left leg where the thigh joined the buttock. After several months, the pain was traveling down the length of her leg, and she was unable to perform her job. The hospital took an MRI, and concluded that the disc between L4 and L5 was protruding, and that this disc impinged on the sciatic nerve and caused her pain. She was recommended to have a discectomy.

She was put on three months' disability leave, during which time she tried six or seven alternative disciplines, none of which worked. During this brief time, her condition so deteriorated that she was unable to walk without assistance.

To cheer her up, one of her friends took her to view a new housing development, thinking that it would be fun to check out the décor of the model homes. One of them had a staircase that Denise was unable to climb, so she sat in the living room looking pained and miserable. The re-altor who was showing the properties inquired after her problem, and hearing it was sciatica, recommended that Denise come see me.

Her sacrum was severely twisted, and pressing S2 elicited terrific pain. I untwisted the sacrum, realigned it, and applied qi to the nerve running out of S2. In two weeks, after two treatments, Denise was almost pain-free, and in a month, she had returned to work with only occasional twinges of pain. Her pain left her completely after six weeks.

Ironically, the hospital was unimpressed by her return to work in a healthy condition. Another MRI showed that the disc was still herniated, and so posed a future health risk. Her present condition was considered to be lucky and temporary. They ordered her to have a discectomy or risk losing her job and medical benefits.

Denise, forced to comply, underwent an endoscopic discectomy. It neither helped her nor hurt her. Her sacrum still has a tendency to twist, but this is easily rectified. To the surprise of her colleagues, she quit her hospital job to work in an oncologist's office.

Seasonal Change and Fine-Tuning

The four seasons according to Americans are as follows:

Spring: The time of year when college students run amok in warm places, and more sober citizens enjoy Easter ham or Passover matzoh.

Summer: The time of year when everybody goes on vacation and barbecues in the backyard.

Autumn: A boring stretch of time redeemed only by Halloween and Thanksgiving.

Winter: The coldest part of the year, but filled with holidays and the thrill of g-force speeds as we streak downhill over snow.

Few of us believe that the change of seasons exerts a physiological effect on the body. After all, thanks to thermal technology, we can live and work at a constant temperature throughout the year. New Zealand and Chile provide the Northern Hemisphere with summer fruits and vegetables during our winter months, and I have no doubt that we reciprocate the favor during their winter months. Refrigerators and freezers preserve food well beyond their natural life span. Man-made fibers resist the winter cold with as little weight as summer cottons. Clean drinking water is piped into our homes year-round, and we do not have to contend with seasonal droughts or floods for the precious fluid. The length of each day is unvarying thanks to electric lighting. We have just as long a workday during the "short" days of winter as during the "long" days of summer. Neither scorching heat nor arctic blasts prevents us from socializing with our friends thanks to well-equipped automobiles. Movie theaters, playhouses, sports arenas, and other places of amusement and entertainment offer us diversion throughout the year.

The list of devices, techniques, and facilities to baffle and defeat the environmental changes of the seasons goes on and on. And yet . . .

Human life was conducted in caves and mud huts for much longer than it has been conducted in centrally heated condos and tract homes with all the modern conveniences.

Put simply, we have not yet evolved into our contemporary living spaces.

You may revel in the fact that you are a Homo sapiens with a university degree and a six-figure income, but physiologically, you are strictly Cro-Magnon, and as such, you are susceptible to all the physiological seasonal changes as your uneducated forebears.

There are actually only two primary seasonally induced changes, but each of these induces smaller changes throughout the body. The body is always adapting/fine-tuning itself to the subtle changes produced by season change.

The two primary changes are, of course, tension and relaxation.

The body is in a constant state of flux as it expands and contracts. It expands (relaxes) in the warm and hot months, and contracts (tenses) in the cool and cold months. There will be as much as an inch difference in your height between the hot and cold seasons.

The body tenses from the feet upward and relaxes from the head downward. You may visualize a wave starting from the soles of your feet and working its way slowly upward, and then, reaching the crown of your head, beginning its descent to the ground. The wave never ceases from the moment of birth until the moment of death.

The body does not begin to adapt to the season when the season changes, but well before so that it enters the season fully prepared for the environmental change.

So, for example, the body begins its change for winter in late August or early September. The body is always one step ahead of the season.

AUTUMN CHANGES (LATE AUGUST TO MID-OCTOBER)

The body needs to contract: skin, hair, teeth, and internal organs all begin to tense. However, we place demands on our bodies in the form of activities that hinder the contracting process. We work just as long hours; we still attend PTA meetings; we maintain an active schedule to fulfill duties and obligations.

In order to promote and facilitate the contracting process, the body will become "tired." We do not feel as energetic as usual, and this forces us to cut back our activities. This tiredness is manifested by tension in T1–4, and weakness in L3 and L4. If the body cannot obtain rest by means of this tiredness, it will next resort to catching colds.

The ankles begin to tighten and stiffen at this time. It is important to rotate the ankles in order to keep them flexible.

The sweat glands, hitherto wide open, begin to close in order to protect the skin. The skin itself begins to tighten as if "battening down the hatches" against the cold of winter. This battening-down process accelerates as the air becomes cooler and drier. Women frequently get dry, flaky skin. The dryness begins at the shins and calves, and progresses up the body to the scalp.

The female pelvis tenses and contracts. When women get an autumn cold or feel tired, this may lead to menstrual irregularity and/or lower backache.

As the body contracts, the pain of old wounds and blows may resurface, and muscle ache, rheumatic-like pain, and other aches and pains arise.

Small children are prone to earaches and nosebleeds at this time.

The stomach contracts; however, most people continue eating the same quantities of food as during summer. This can lead to more tiredness, even to fatigue as the stomach struggles to cope.

PRE-WINTER CHANGES (LATE OCTOBER TO EARLY DECEMBER)

The body's contraction is almost complete. The spine has now contracted, and the scalp begins to contract. The body has a tendency to become dehydrated. Plenty of liquids, especially warm liquids such as soups and broths, help ease the body into winter.

If the lips and sides of the mouth become dry, this is a sure sign of dehydration. The body will do all it can to retain water, and so will become bloated if liquid intake is not increased. This bloating is usually seen in women in one of the thighs. It will be larger than the other.

T11 will become stiff and painful if dehydration persists. Middle-back pain can be alleviated by drinking a lot of water.

Finally, a lack of water at this time will lead to stiff shoulders.

The hamstrings become tight and tender to the touch. It is good to give direct qi to the hamstrings if you feel stiffness there.

WINTER CHANGES (EARLY DECEMBER TO MID-JANUARY)

The body has closed up; contraction is complete. The skin is tight and has lost a lot of moisture. The waist and hips are also tight, and so the body loses some flexibility. Twisting and turning from side to side are not as easy as in the period of warmth. One arm is likely to feel dull and the shoulder blade on that side may get tight, even a bit achy. The lumbar vertebrae are frequently tight, and the muscles alongside them may become tender to the touch.

EARLY-SPRING CHANGES (MID-JANUARY TO MID-FEBRUARY)

The body begins to loosen in anticipation of spring. The loosening process begins at the top of the head and works its way slowly downward. You can feel the scalp relax from the crown of the head to the lower back of the head, and the skin of the scalp and face becomes more moist and oily. Following this, the cervical vertebrae begin to loosen. This expansion should be encouraged. This can be done by letting warm water run over the back of the neck when showering. It is also useful to place a hot compress on the sides of the bridge of the nose for two or three minutes daily.

SPRING CHANGES (MID-FEBRUARY TO MID-MARCH)

The cervical vertebrae will have relaxed by now. It is time for the thoracic vertebrae to follow. In early March, the lumbar vertebrae and pelvis will loosen, so that the body will be flexible and relaxed for the warmth of spring.

As the thoracic vertebrae begin to loosen, people commonly experience stiff shoulders or pain in the upper back. In extreme cases, upper back spasms occur. It is not uncommon for T6 to twist, and this leads to problems with digestion, most notably acid reflux (heartburn).

As the head, neck, and upper back begin to relax, the mind, which has been fairly tranquil during the cold months, begins to buzz with activity. It may become filled with repetitive, annoying thoughts or hints of thoughts. (A healthy mind indulges in flights of fancy or imaginative fantasies.) The sensation of anxiety is not uncommon at this time, and this feeling leads to shortness of breath. I have been told that this is the peak season for suicides. Feelings of anxiety or repetitive morbid thoughts should pass as the weather turns warmer, and the body is naturally induced to sleep more deeply.

As the thoracic vertebrae relax, female skin may blemish easily and lose some of its natural moisture. It is a good time of year to add body oil to your bathwater.

March is the most important time of year for the female reproductive system. There may be a tender, stationary lump in one of the breasts, located on the side of the breast where it meets the rib cage. It is easy to check for this lump by lying on the back, and feeling along the side of the breast with the middle, ring, and little fingers of the opposite hand. This lump will pass as the season changes. This breast usually corresponds to the working ovary that month. It is a useful means of ascertaining the working ovary in order to keep track of the menstrual cycle.

Women should give themselves, or receive from others, direct qi to the resting ovary in order to ensure a smooth and regular menstrual cycle for the rest of the warm weather period.

As the ankles begin to relax from the tension of winter, they may be weak and unstable. Be sure to give them plenty of stretching exercise to impart strength and flexibility.

EARLY-SUMMER CHANGES (MID-MARCH TO EARLY JUNE)

Summer is the season of peak expansion. The spine lengthens to full extension, and a person normally "grows" a half inch to an inch in height. The shoulders, lower back, and hips tend to twist in the direction of the individual's dominant side. The result is often a weak or aching lower back. Twisting the body by looking over your shoulder should be done several times a day as a corrective to this natural twist.

The body enlarges despite a smaller appetite. Weight gain of two to four pounds is not uncommon during summer. The body stabilizes itself by lowering its center of gravity slightly. Weight is directed downward, toward the ground.

The body's metabolic rate increases. Body cleansing—through the digestive system, urinary tract, and the skin—is performed faster at this time of year. External stimuli are felt more keenly, as are emotional stimuli. Joy, sorrow, optimism, anger, and other emotions seem more intense at this time of year. There is a tendency to act on impulse, and it is good to think something through before putting the impulse into action.

The quality of sleep will improve from early May. Sleep will become deeper and more refreshing. When this happens, the mind will relax and anxious thoughts will pass.

SUMMER CHANGES (EARLY JUNE TO LATE AUGUST)

There is a tendency for the pulmonary system to weaken. Be aware of your breathing and if you are feeling satisfied by the fullness of your breath.

Putting qi directly into the top back of the head between Head Point Numbers 3 and 5 will strengthen the pulmonary system, increase appetite, and prepare the body for a smooth transition into autumn.

If the elbow joint(s) becomes stiff during summertime, hold the elbow in the palm of your hand and give direct qi. Anyone who has ever dinged his elbow knows about the existence of the "funny bone." This is a nerve cluster at the elbow joint. This is the point into which you put your direct qi.

Biorhythms

Our bodies are in a state of unceasing flux and motion both microscopically and macroscopically. Our hearts beat, our lungs respire, our skin expands and contracts, and all the atomic and subatomic particles that constitute our frame zoom all about our living autobahn. Our bodies also come equipped with an unceasing rhythm that naturally tenses and relaxes us. In the world of qi, this rhythm is called a "tide," and our minds and bodies are always moving between "flood tide" and "ebb tide." You may think of the former as "active" and the latter as "passive." For those of a Far Eastern bent, think "yang" and "yin."

The tides are like the Russian folk dolls that live one inside the other, each becoming progressively smaller. Our largest tide is birth and death. We are born at flood tide, and die at ebb tide, though there is a sudden and powerful transition to flood tide at the exact moment of death. Each of us has a lengthy rhythm cycle of varying duration. Mine is nine years; that of my wife is seven years. The next rhythm durations become progressively shorter: a yearly rhythm, a monthly rhythm, a weekly rhythm, and a daily rhythm. We are most aware of our monthly rhythm.

A pregnant woman goes into the active flood tide from the moment of conception until approximately ten days before labor begins, at which time she goes into the passive ebb tide. The fetus is in ebb tide until the mother swings into ebb tide, at which time it changes to flood tide.

The woman is physically responsible for the welfare of herself and her fetus for the term of the pregnancy, and so stays at flood tide. The fetus is dominated by the mother's qi and physicality, and so stays at ebb tide for nine months.

When labor begins, Nature has seen to it that the baby fights its way into the world through the birth canal, and this requires it to be in the active flood tide. At the same time, the mother must relax so that her pelvis opens to maximum width in order to allow the baby to come out easily. She goes into the passive ebb tide.

At the moment of birth, the baby once again lapses into ebb tide, and the mother, faced with feeding and nurturing a helpless creature, changes into flood tide. It takes the new mother about six weeks to return to her characteristic flux between ebb and flood tides.

The physical and mental characteristics of flood tide are as follows: the face is firm, compact, and has good color and sheen; the hair is firm and "works well"; you do not need as much sleep time or food to function at full energy; the memory is sharp; you do not forget or lose things; you tend to be forward looking and even optimistic.

The physical and mental characteristics of ebb tide are as follows: the face is pallid, loose, puffy, and seems wider than usual; the hair is soft, lank, and does not "work well"; the palms tend to be moist or sweaty; it takes more sleep and food to function at full tilt; you tend to be absentminded, and forget or lose things; your outlook is past and present-oriented, and life does not seem to present many opportunities.

The tides manifest themselves in a pulse just above the navel. This pulse rate corresponds to that found on the wrist. Having accessed your qi, place two fingers one inch above and one inch to the left of the navel, and see if you feel the pulse. Then try placing your fingers one inch above and one inch to the right of the navel.

A pulse on the left indicates flood tide, a pulse on the right indicates ebb tide. The pulse may travel further than an inch from the left or right of the navel. The further from the navel the pulse is found, the more pronounced the degree of the tide.

Another way to ascertain tide is as follows: with the person lying on his back, watch carefully as he inhales and exhales. If the inhalation is longer than the exhalation, he is in a state of flood tide. A longer exhalation indicates ebb tide.

Doing *kiryū* on a regular basis will keep your body's natural rhythm moving smoothly between the two tides.

CASE HISTORY

My wife, Therese, was feeling and behaving uncharacteristically. Her hair wouldn't do what she wanted it to; she was constipated; she was moody; she slept and slept, yet could not shake off a feeling of tiredness; food did not taste as good as it used to; and she had trouble concentrating and frequently dropped things.

This state of affairs continued for a couple of months, and although it was annoying, we were only slightly worried that it indicated a deeper problem.

Kayoko Matsuura, on the other hand, was overjoyed.

"Your biorhythm is on a seven-year cycle, and you are now at the lowest point of it," she chirped with delight. "You could come out of it naturally, but that would take months. Why wait? Let's start you climbing back into flood tide today."

Mrs. Matsuura worked on Therese for twenty minutes, and then declared that she was out of the woods.

We left Mrs. Matsuura's house and began walking toward the train station when all of a sudden Therese said she felt tired. She had been saying that for two months, so I did not pay any attention, but continued walking. I had gone about thirty feet when I realized that I was walking alone. Therese had fallen down in the road, dead asleep.

I could not revive her. I half-carried, half-dragged her to the station and pushed her onto a train. She slept the entire two-hour trip to our station. I then had to carry her home. I dropped her on the bed, and she continued sleeping for eighteen hours.

When she awoke, she raced to the toilet where she ensconced herself for two hours of almost continuous relief. With the final flush, she returned to bed and slept another eight hours.

The next day when she woke, her hair was working well and all of her lovable characteristics had returned.

She has passed through two more seven-year cycles since then. Her low point was never as pronounced as that first experience, as a result of applying qi to the pulse on her right side, and doing *kiryū* twice a day during that period.

Sleep

Sleep, that knits up the ravelled sleave of care,
The death of each day's life, sore labour's bath,
Balm of hurt minds, great nature's second course,
Chief nourisher in life's feast.

—SHAKESPEARE, *Macbeth, II, ii*

Thomas Young, less long-winded than Shakespeare, called sleep "Tired Nature's sweet restorer."

Sleep is not a body system, yet, as the above quotations indicate, sleep has such an influence on all our other body systems that it makes sense to include it in the chapter on body systems.

We all know that a good night's sleep can make us feel like a million bucks, while a bad night's sleep leaves us feeling like death warmed over. Poor sleeping makes it difficult to concentrate, leaves us feeling grumpy or short-tempered, diminishes our appetite for food and fun, and generally affects our outlook on life itself.

Quality of sleep is related to quality of breath. When you breathe deeply, you sleep deeply. When your breath is shallow, your sleep is shallow. A vigorous life in which tension and relaxation are nicely balanced creates vitality, and vitality is essential to quality of breath. Cares and worries reduce vitality to the point of effacement and upset the balance of tension and relaxation.

The fact that worry can inhibit sleep demonstrates the connection between the activity of the brain and the functioning of the lungs (pulmonary system). The intimacy of this connection cannot be overstated, and yet it passes unnoticed by most people though it manifests itself right before them almost daily.

Consider feelings of anxiety. They produce shortness of breath. Extreme anxiety can produce hyperventilation, a condition in which you breathe so rapidly but so shallowly that you can faint. Fear and panic (not just in emergency situations, but also arising from phobias) also induce shortness of breath. In fact, at frightening moments, many people actually catch and hold their breath, causing the body to tremble and sweat, finally leaving them "gasping with fear."

On the other hand, moments of beauty and joy can also affect our breath. When we behold a glorious sight we "gasp for joy" or give a "gasp of delight." Thinking that something bad is about to befall us and finding out that our fears were, after all, groundless produces a "sigh of relief."

Regret and disappointment can also make us sigh. Long ago, it was customary for young men to demonstrate that they were in love by sighing at regular intervals. Parting lovers were always given to sighing.

In short, our thoughts are given instant substance by means of the pulmonary system. Thus, when we consider sleep disorders, we must also consider other mind/pulmonary connections, such as anxiety and asthma. Most cases of asthma have psychological factors involved. An asthmatic who feels an attack coming on will reach for his inhaler. Just feeling it snug in his hand will prevent the attack. Should he remember that he left it in his car or at home, the attack will begin.

In the world of diagnosis by qi, anxiety and asthma present the same symptoms as sleep disorders, and the treatment for all three is the same.

The difference between them is that sleep disorders and anxiety may be induced by seasonal change, while asthma never is, except insofar as the asthma is related to pollen count or other environmental factors.

Prolonged light or poor sleep produces a number of physical phenomena.

1. The scalp becomes loose, particularly on the right side. If you try to pinch and hold the skin of a good sleeper at the base of the skull corresponding to the location of C2, the flesh will be too tight to grasp. Conversely, you will be able to pinch and hold a lot of skin at the same site on a poor sleeper. The more skin you can pinch, the worse the sleep disorder. If you can get a good amount of flesh between your fingers an inch above the C2 point, it indicates waking two to three times per night with trouble returning to sleep. Grasping flesh as high as Head Point Number 5 indicates insomnia.

2. The rib cage contracts, usually on one side rather than on both sides. The intercostal muscles (the muscles between the ribs that patrons of barbecue enjoy as spareribs) become tense and contract. This shortens the rib cage.

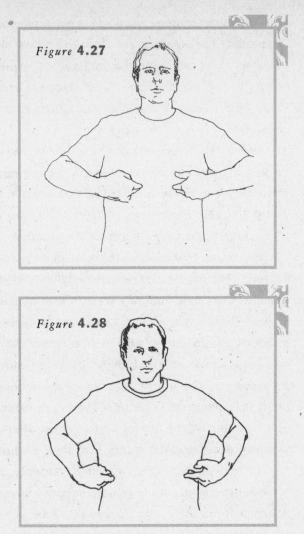

Figure **4.27**

Figure **4.28**

To determine the length of your rib cage, stand in front of a mirror. Place your fingers, palms upward, in the center of your chest under your rib cage. Follow the line of the rib cage to the sides of your body. You can see if both sides are in or out of alignment (see Figures 4.27 and 4.28).

A sleep disorder will produce a misalignment of between one and two inches, meaning that one side is much shorter than the other. The lung capacity of the affected side will be diminished, resulting in shallow breathing. This perpetuates the cycle of poor sleep.

3. The first four thoracic vertebrae (T1, T2, T3, T4) become very tense, even falling out of alignment. (In the case of chronic anxiety, T4 becomes as hard as stone and frequently protrudes.) Pulmonary function is inhibited when these vertebrae lose so much flexibility that they are unable to perform to their full potential. Moreover, when these vertebrae are tense and/or misaligned, the upper back tends to become stiff and painful. There is frequently a band of pain running across the upper back, which becomes an impediment to sleep.

4. The coccyx (commonly called the tailbone) goes out of alignment. The coccyx is, in most people, comprised of four bones. Poor sleep causes the coccyx to twist or the bones to fall out of alignment, frequently producing sciatica. This is particularly true in the case of women. Men do not suffer from misaligned coccyx as frequently as women do.

5. The Achilles tendons become very stiff, and the ankles lose their flexibility. The Achilles tendons are closely related to mental activity. Stiff Achilles tendons indicate tension in the mind as manifested by repetitive thoughts, needless fears and worries, anxiety, or sensory overstimulation. Loose Achilles tendons indicate just the opposite—an easygoing, relaxed outlook and thought process.

6. The liver becomes overworked and tired when a poor sleep pattern emerges. Our breath performs a double function; it nourishes and cleanses. Obviously, if our breath is shallow, then the nourishing and cleansing activities of the oxygen in the blood are not performed sufficiently well. What you put in your mouth to nourish you must be released by the body after the nutrients have been removed. Failure to do so will result in the body's being poisoned. There are a number of ways to cleanse, one of which is through the breath: in with oxygen, out with carbon dioxide. The liver is perhaps the premier cleansing organ of the body, and it will pick up the slack of other organs, including the lungs.

    The result of diminished lung capacity and shallowness of breath is that liver function actually declines when a person sleeps poorly.

TREATING SLEEP DISORDERS

The Heart of the Hand
Place your right thumb over the heart of the receiver's right hand, and send qi until you feel the bone below your thumb "soften."

The Head
The receiver should be lying on his stomach, head turned to his right. The giver stands at the receiver's head. The giver places the heart of his right hand on Head Point

Number 5, and the heart of his left hand on Head Point Number 1 (see Figure 4.29).

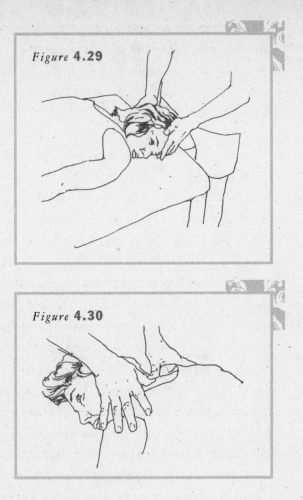

Figure **4.29**

Figure **4.30**

The right hand is active, and the left hand is passive. Send qi from your right hand though the head to your left hand. People whose bodies crave sleep will literally suck the qi right out of your hand. It is not so much a question of sending qi as it is just holding still and letting the receiver's body take as much as it needs. The heart of your right hand will grow warm, and you will feel a flow of qi with your left hand.

When the warmth of the right hand reaches a plateau and begins to subside, the flow of qi to the left hand will also subside. At this time, exhale slowly and, as you do so, slowly remove your hands from the receiver's head.

The First Four Thoracic Vertebrae

Still standing at the receiver's head, place your right thumb on the T1 vertebra, and then cover it with your left thumb (see Figure 4.30). T1 is just below the protruding C7 and is the first vertebra that does not turn together with the head.

Send qi with both of your thumbs into T1 for a minute. You will feel the bone begin to "soften." The bone does not really soften, but you have the feeling that it is not as spiky as it was, but has gotten softer and rounder. Go next to T2 and T3, concluding with T4.

When you have finished putting qi directly into each of the four vertebrae, return to T1. Place your thumbs on either side of the vertebra. There should be a groove

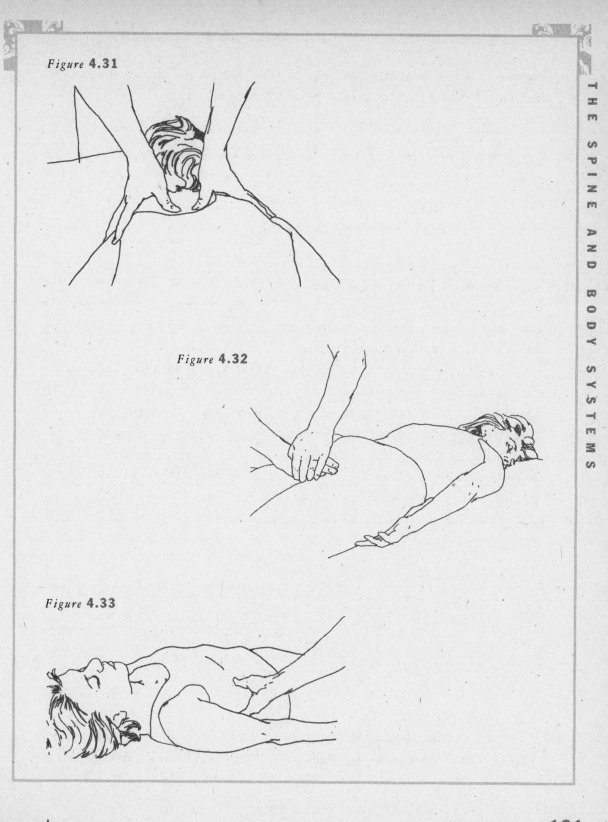

Figure **4.31**

Figure **4.32**

Figure **4.33**

running alongside the spinal cord (see Figure 4.31). Send qi with your thumbs into the points for a minute. Then repeat the procedure with T2 through T4.

The Coccyx

Move to the receiver's left side. Place your right hand directly over the coccyx and cover it with your left hand. Put qi into the coccyx for a little over a minute (see Figure 4.32).

Following these three procedures, the receiver turns over on to his back.

The Rib Cage

Let us assume you have already determined which side of the rib cage is contracted. If you have not done so, it is easy to do. Follow the method given earlier (see page 118), but, as the receiver is supine rather than standing, you will have to use your thumbs and not your index, middle, and ring fingers.

Stand at the receiver's side. Place your right thumb between two ribs along the side of the body (see Figure 4.33). You will be able to feel a gap between the ribs, although, when the ribs are contracted, the gap is not nearly as wide as when the rib cage is open. Send qi into the gap for a minute.

Go to the opposite side of the receiver, and place your right hand over the spot where you gave qi, and cover it with your left hand. Lifting the rib cage gently toward yourself, send qi in for about thirty seconds (see Figure 4.34).

Check the size of the rib cage once again to make sure the contracted side has expanded and is relaxed.

The Achilles Tendons

Stand or sit at the receiver's feet. Hold the feet with your hands so that the Achilles tendons rest on the hearts of your hands (see Figure 4.35). Send qi into the tendons. One tendon should feel colder to you than the other. When it has "warmed up," you may move to the next stage. If you do not feel a cold or warmth, put qi into the tendons for just over a minute.

The Liver

The liver is located directly below the rib cage on the right side. To locate it, place your right hand on the rib cage, and slide it down until the left side of your hand is no

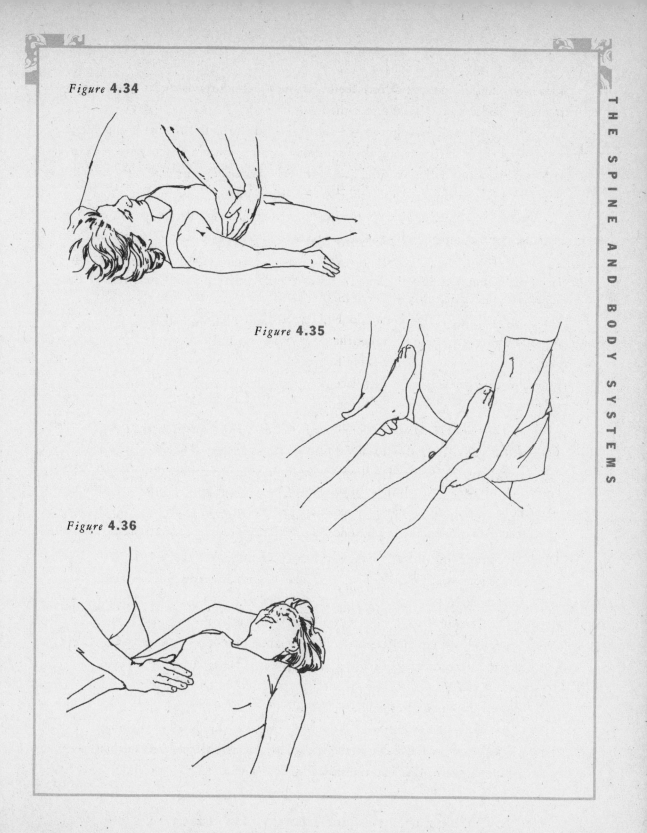

Figure **4.34**

Figure **4.35**

Figure **4.36**

longer on the rib cage, but directly below it and touching the last rib. Your hand is now over the liver (see Figure 4.36).

With your right hand spread over the liver, send qi into the liver with your whole hand. After about thirty seconds, the liver should grow warm and you may even feel energy swirling about within it. After about a minute, the liver under your hand actually feels like it is expanding or "plumping up." Continue giving qi for another minute.

When you finish and slowly remove your hand on an exhalation, you might notice that the abdominal cavity has become rounder and sleeker than it had been.

The treatment for sleep disorders, asthma, and anxiety is now complete. However, you may want to do paired *kiryū* to complete the treatment and promote the changes you have already made.

Daily treatments should produce beneficial results within five days.

CASE HISTORY

My mother, Marty, suffered from chronic sciatica for more than two years. The full story of how Kayoko Matsuura healed her may be read elsewhere, and so here I will present only the salient features of her story.

X-rays revealed that Marty had no discs between her lumbar vertebrae. All the physicians and chiropractors who viewed the X-rays ruled conclusively that, without discs to mediate between them, the vertebrae were impinging on the sciatic nerve. Only a laminectomy to fuse the vertebrae together into a shotgun wedding of alignment could provide relief, they believed.

Kayoko Matsuura listened to Marty's sad tale and then had her lie down on her stomach. After a minute of sending qi into her head and spine, she had Marty turn over, and she put her hands on Marty's liver and rib cage.

"You are a poor sleeper," she remarked, "You don't look forward to sleep and are not refreshed by sleep."

Marty was astonished. "How do you know?" she asked. In the small circles she moved in she was well known as a terrible sleeper, but she had no idea that her reputation extended as far as Japan.

"Your body told me," Mrs. Matsuura replied matter-of-factly, and proceeded to work on Marty.

After two treatments, Marty was told that she was structurally perfect, and that the sciatica would leave her in a short time. Marty was ecstatic and ran off to a local hospital in Tokyo to have X-rays taken to confirm this diagnosis.

Alas, the X-rays were an exact match of those she had brought to Japan from the United States. Marty was crushed and scheduled another appointment with Mrs. Matsuura.

"You told me that I was structurally perfect," she complained, "but nothing has changed in my lower back."

"Of course not," Mrs. Matsuura replied, "there was never anything wrong with your lower back. Why would I work on it?"

Marty was baffled and frustrated.

Mrs. Matsuura calmly explained her approach to Marty's cure.

"I noticed at once that you are a poor sleeper. I naturally thought that your coccyx would be out of alignment, and indeed it was. You have no discs between your lumbars, it's true, but the muscles are supporting and moving them nicely, and they are not giving you any trouble. The trouble was with the coccyx. Did you ever have X-rays taken of your coccyx?"

Marty shook her head.

"I thought not." Mrs. Matsuura turned away, terminating the conversation. But Marty, still baffled, asked for a fuller explanation. Mrs. Matsuura explained the relationship between sleep and the integrity of the coccyx in women, and then proceeded to tell Marty that she had straightened her coccyx, opened the right side of the rib cage, stimulated her liver, and sent a lot of qi into her sleep points.

Marty left the clinic only fifty percent convinced by Mrs. Matsuura's assessment of her situation. Yet she soon began sleeping soundly, and her sciatica disappeared. She learned how to do *kiryū* in order to maintain her structural integrity by herself.

That was in 1984, and she has never been bothered by sciatica since.

CHAPTER 5

Pregnancy And Childbirth

Qi for Two

Thirty years ago there were mothers and fathers. There still are, but there are also "partners" and "consorts" and "significant others" and "surrogate" mothers, and conception without intercourse for couples and single women.

I have written this chapter with the idea that yours is a wanted pregnancy and, trepidation about pregnancy to one side, you are looking forward to having a child as a welcome addition to your life. And more, that another person is actively involved in the process and is as desirous of the child as you are.

The word "partner" lacks the nuance of intimacy for me, and I would like to think of the act of creation as arising from at least an emotional intimacy. The word "father" may not apply to all readers.

I have chosen to call the person with whom the mother is having her child (or sharing her pregnancy) the "parent." This word strikes me as having forceful, active overtones; a real stake in the process of creation and beyond. Thus, though the linkage may initially jar through unfamiliarity, I will refer to the expecting couple as parent and mother.

Thoughts on Pregnancy

Pregnancy does not ask anything of the female body that it is not able to perform with ease. In fact, since women were physiologically created for pregnancy and have been going through "wardrobe fittings" monthly for their moment on stage, the act of pregnancy should stimulate the female body to the very peak of health and physical well-being.

Yet, the pregnant woman today is placed in an unenviable position. Her condition, if not treated as an outright disease, is certainly not treated as a positive state of health. The OB/GYN assumes the role of primary health-care provider, while the mother is treated as an unreliable incubator that requires frequent monitoring. She is admonished as to what to eat and drink, and how to walk and exercise. She comes to rely on the stethoscope and ultrasound to locate her baby at lengthy intervals, and plays classical music in the hope of improving its IQ *in utero.* In a very real sense, she is kept apart from the life within her.

Then there is a powerful psychological factor at work. That is, the condition of pregnancy is presented as a locked room in which a woman is incarcerated for nine months. She is alone with her fetus. No one can help. The parent is asked to be understanding and caring, but it is assumed that there is little he can do for the mother other than humor her and lavish her with sympathy. The success or failure of the enterprise is on her shoulders.

The pregnant woman is thus confronted with a paradox: her health and the health of her fetus are dependent on a second party, while she feels that physically and psychologically her pregnancy is a solo venture.

What is more, she knows from books or hearsay that she is fated to experience some or all of the following: pregnancy rhinitis, morning sickness, lower back pain, leg cramps, and worse. Even if these do not occur, she is told stories and anecdotes about the pain of labor and marathon childbirth experiences.

No wonder many women are anxious about pregnancy or experience it with discomfort.

The above view of pregnancy is wrong, and it is unhealthy because it is wrong, and wrong because it is unhealthy.

Pregnancy is a potential state of superb health that, with proper guidance, can fill the woman with a glowing sense of wellness and vigor. I maintain that the mother can and should be the primary health-care giver to her fetus, and that pregnancy is far from being, of its very nature, a solitary affair.

The mother's body is constantly changing during pregnancy. This means physical changes that can be observed and hormonal changes that cannot. The regular application of qi will make the changes smooth and painless. Qi will keep the pelvis and lower body flexible, which is vitally important for having an easy natural birth. By means of qi, you will be able to talk to your fetus. Both the mother and the parent can locate the child, get to know the child, entertain the child, and "educate" the child *in utero*. Simply put, the child becomes accessible to you, and you both can truly get to know your child from the moment of conception, and have the baby cooperate at the birth.

A final thought: You are not the first to have a child, and if you are the last, the human race is doomed to extinction. You are now an active member of the vital continuum of history. What is important is to enjoy the state of maternity. That means, with hands-on qi and your own goodwill, raising your baby *ab ovo,* from the egg.

The Baby Palace

You're pregnant! It's official! Congratulations!

You have just fulfilled Step One of your biological destiny.

You may believe you were born to be wild or to be an actress or a Wall Street tycoon or the wife of Prince Charming. With all due respect, you were born to propagate the human race. Everything beyond that is gravy.

Unfortunately, from the moment of your child's conception, there are many shrill, even strident voices competing for your attention, each of whose pronouncements sows a seed of worry or unease.

Eat this! Don't eat that! Drink this! Don't drink that! Have you started a college fund yet? I didn't get a good night's sleep for the first three years after Junior was born! You have to go to the gym! You'll ruin yourself if you go to the gym now! I was nine hours in labor! and so on.

Collectively, these competing voices produce stress, tension, and even dread. Your mind and body tense, which inhibits the natural physiological progress of the pregnancy in which the body easily adjusts itself to its new state. The voices' prophecies induce the unhealthy state they purport to warn you against.

To return to my original statement: Congratulations! You have just fulfilled Step One of your biological destiny.

You were born with a full complement of eggs. From the onset of menarche, your body has been preparing to get pregnant. The entire rhythm of your life has been dominated by your body's desire to conceive. Every month, your body has produced an egg or two, and constructed a cozy nest in which to fertilize, nourish, and protect the next generation. And every month, when the egg and nest go past their prime unused, your body cleanses itself to prepare a nest for the next egg.

You might think of it as your body diligently and persistently preparing a special room for a special guest. And when the guest finally arrives, your body is glad. Think of the "Be Our Guest" extravaganza sequence in the animated Disney movie *Beauty and the Beast,* and you will have a pretty clear idea of how your body feels about your new guest.

In Chinese and Japanese, the word for "womb" means "baby palace." I find this a lovely image. The palace is large and clean and (usually) houses a single ruler. All things necessary to maintain a comfortable life are provided free of charge: food, air, water, warmth, and indoor plumbing. No wonder at some time or other we all wish to return there.

The palace is a place of security, "sounds and sweet airs that give delight and hurt not." The baby does not so much hear your voice as experience it. He is enveloped by energy and vibrations within the palace walls.

What is more, the palace expands at the same rate as the baby. There is no need to add on a wing or convert the turret into a closet. Nor is there any need for demolition once your ruler/guest has departed the palace.

In contrast, the English word "hysteria" derives from the Greek word for "womb," as the condition was thought to occur from disturbances in the uterus. A newly expecting mother may well be driven to that condition by unnecessary and unwholesome concern for her well-being. The state of pregnancy is not a disturbance in the uterus. Think of a *baby palace,* and relax.

Pregnancy, then, is the most natural thing in the world. It follows that, since a woman is created to house the next generation, her body will naturally grow and strengthen to accommodate the changes caused by the arrival of her guest. So, from the time you are informed that you have conceived, you should consciously think of your physical state as follows: **Pregnancy and childbirth are fundamental to the human organism, and Nature has seen to it that both be as simple as possible.**

If you are unable to enjoy your pregnancy, you should at least be prepared to be an interested and active part of what is perhaps the most interesting experience available to human beings.

Qi and the Pregnant Woman

My wife, Therese, is also a qi practitioner. Within a week of learning she was pregnant, I felt a change in her energy when she worked on me. It had become stronger and more incisive, yet it had a soothing quality to it. Although I physically felt this change, I ascribed it to wishful thinking on my part. No doubt my delight at her pregnancy had colored my senses, and led me to feel what was not, in fact, there.

Three weeks into her pregnancy, when she and I were still the only ones who knew, Therese's patients began to feel the change. Not only did they comment on the intensity of her energy, but noted that her treatments, usually effective, had become much more so and took less time. What normally took thirty minutes to change in the body could now be done in ten. So I had not been deluded by joy!

Her energy continued to strengthen and refine itself as her pregnancy progressed. She followed the regimen to be detailed below, and found her energy attaining a remarkable ability to calm and heal. Our business was never so good as patients became quite addicted to her touch and clamored for more. As did I. The more selfish of us would have liked her pregnancy to continue for years.

Following the birth of our son, her energy returned to its original quality. She lost her superpowers with motherhood. The state of pregnancy had transformed her original qi into something more vital and potent than either of us had imagined possible. This is true for all pregnant women. Why this is, I cannot say for sure. There are several possible reasons.

The natural energy (qi) of a pregnant woman does not double in the case of a single pregnancy or treble in the case of bearing twins. Her energy grows exponentially, out of all proportion to the fact that she is now two or three people rather than one. Not only that, but her energy becomes a potent force for health and healing. It is literally a nurturing energy.

It seems to me that the female body contains a mass of latent power that does not come into play until the organism becomes pregnant. This is like Pavarotti's using his voice to sing only nursery rhymes, or the space shuttle's being used to go to and from the market—the greater part of the potential is wasted. The female body was created to reproduce in quantity, and it is at the moment of conception that the latent energy rises to the surface. It is like striking an underground oil pocket and producing a gusher. That is why a pregnant woman's energy is not just a matter of her energy plus that of her child. It is that her qi has surged to its fullest, strongest, and ripest.

When, in addition to this outpouring of healthy energy, the mother's feelings for her child are loving, the healing and nurturing qualities of her qi are even further enhanced. It is, therefore, an excellent time for the pregnant woman to use her "gift" for herself and others. Applying her qi to remove pain, aid in healing cuts and bruises, relaxing herself and her partner, and so on will be more effective and beneficial than at any other time of her life. The procedures given in Chapter 4 are doubly effective when a pregnant woman applies her qi.

I am always eager to give energy to, and receive energy from, a pregnant woman. Because qi always re-creates itself, I never feel tired or weary after giving qi treatments. Working on a pregnant woman, however, is one of the most energizing and exhilarating experiences possible. I feel as if I could carry on for hours. My energy feeds off hers as it were, and gains in strength and intensity.

It is true that the mother's energy returns to its original state following childbirth. However, the nurturing quality of that energy has been intensified through nine months of co-occupancy of a single space, and the love the new mother feels for her newborn.

The First Trimester

THE BUN IN THE OVEN

As a man—the parent—I found that for me the highlight of Therese's pregnancy for me was my involvement and daily participation. That participation was due largely to qi treatments that allowed me to do the following:

1. provide physical comfort and a tangible sense of intimacy to Therese.
2. establish a rapport and an intimacy with my son.
3. share in the prenatal activities of discipline and education.

And to the benefit of us both, my active participation provided us with endless hours of happy conversation as *we* talked about the progress of *our* child. Without giving hands-on treatment, I would have been ignorant of what was going on in the womb, and baby conversation would have been one-sided.

So let's get the parent actively involved from Day One.

The first thing for you and the parent to do is give the baby a working name. The name is not intended to be permanent, but is to be used only as long as the child is *in utero.*

Your child is a work in progress, and the name can be changed at any time. In fact, as you get to know your child *in utero,* you may change the name according to the latest developments in the child's behavior. Naming the child is simply a fun way to relate to the child, and an effective means of transmitting qi to it because a name is specific and calls forth all sorts of associations and passions.

Many, if not most, mothers and parents call the fetus Baby. I have nothing against calling the child Baby. I do, however, feel it lacks memorable intimacy. After all, most partners have nicknames for each other, even if they are only Sweetheart and Darling.

It is a little hard to imagine that, as you see your child off to her first day of kindergarten, the two of you will look at each other and say, "Do you remember when we called her Baby?" It will be far more touching to be able to say, "Do you remember when we called her Tadpole?" or some such. Even Qi Baby would be preferable to plain Baby.

By doing qi exercises with your baby, you will get to know certain of his characteristics. Some babies respond to qi by buzzing. Others by wiggling. Others by sending out a tickling sensation. Each has her own response to qi, and this response can provide a fun and descriptive name for the child. Hint: the title of this section is suggestive of a good name.

AWARENESS OF CHILD-REARING

Child-rearing does not begin with birth, but from conception.

I will take up the subject of physical substances entering the fetus later in this chapter. At this juncture, I feel it is imperative to emphasize that all emotions enter the fetus through the blood and body chemistry. Adrenaline rushes into the fetus, as do "poisonous" feelings such as hatred and revenge. The mother and parent need an ongoing awareness of this fact, especially during the first thirteen weeks of pregnancy.

During the first trimester, a woman is more susceptible to the influence of qi than at any other time of her life. She is far more susceptible than a man will ever be. Qi is absorbed and distributed throughout the body to great effect and little waste. Emotions, when translated into qi, are vigorously flushed through the body. Happiness, laughter, merriment, and joy will invigorate and stimulate fetal development. Anxiety, dread, anger, frustration, and hatred will produce the opposite effect. Further, the negative impact on the mother's physical health cannot be overstated.

The fact is, the first thirteen weeks of pregnancy are, psychologically, the most difficult. There are real adjustments to make. As stated earlier, most anecdotes and literature about pregnancy are plain scary. It takes time to learn that they are the exception rather than the rule. The mother may be ambivalent about having a child. The parent may also be ambivalent about his new status, and produce anxiety within the living environment.

If a miscarriage occurs, it is likely to occur within this thirteen-week time frame. The mother will learn this willy-nilly from physician or friend. This knowledge becomes an added, perhaps the paramount, source of anxiety.

The most important element of getting easily and successfully through the first thirteen weeks is to remain tranquil and sedate.

All external problems and worries should be measured against the health of the child, and then a healthy perspective will be achieved.

Besides trying to avoid stress and negative feelings as much as is humanly possible, *in utero* child-rearing is accomplished by (1) direct transmission of qi to the fetus, (2) walking, and (3) consciously including "Bun" in your activities of daily life.

QI FOR TWO

The health of the mother takes priority over that of the fetus during the first thirteen weeks. If the mother is healthy and calm, the fetus will do well.

I wrote above that during the first thirteen weeks the mother is highly sensitive and susceptible to qi. From the moment of conception, the mother's qi has grown and intensified. She is as strong in qi as several people rolled into one. Her qi will grow in strength as the baby grows, but her sudden surge in qi strength is evident from the start. This is a very good time for the mother to use her qi to relax herself, the parent, and to stimulate fetal growth.

Qi should be given directly to the fetus on a daily basis by the mother, the parent or (ideally) both. As each individual's qi has its own characteristics and "flavor," it is ideal for the mother and parent to introduce themselves to their child through qi as early as possible.

Qi can be given to the fetus with either the right hand or with both hands. Do not give qi using only the left hand. The body is bipolar (+/-) like a magnet. The right hand is the conduit for active qi (+), the left for passive qi (-). You should avoid giving your baby only passive qi until after birth.

It is more pleasurable for the mother to give qi with both hands. Lying comfortably on your back, place both hands on your belly just above the pubic bone. This is slightly below the location for giving yourself ovarian qi (see Figure 4.14 on page 95). The fetus will be under there somewhere. He moves from left to right, and right to left. In time, certainly by the end of the fourth week, you will be able to locate the fetus by means of his response to your qi.

Imagine that you are cupping your child within the palms of your hands. You are holding him and keeping him safe and secure.

While giving qi, you should have a constant thought process, like a tape loop, that is rhythmically linked to your breathing. Thoughts should be positive and directed toward the fetus.

During the first month of pregnancy, it is hard to imagine what is inside your belly. However, from the fifth week, you may imagine or visualize a living creature the size of the top joint of your pinkie. That tiny being is living directly beneath your palms when you give qi, and will fit easily into them. Channel your thoughts to your child.

"I am creating a strong, healthy child."

"I am providing Bun with a wonderful environment."

"I am providing each and every life support for Bun."

"I am nourishing my child with qi."

"I am communicating my love to Bun."

Make your thoughts as rhythmic as possible. If your breathing is slow, think slowly. The qi goes into the fetus continually, not only when you exhale. Aligning your thoughts and your breathing creates a strong, steady sensation.

With positive and loving thoughts, you will feel your hands warm up. You may even feel a sharp tingling in the center of your palms that comes and goes. **This is the fetus responding to your qi.** Responses will become stronger and more regular as the baby grows and gets to know your qi.

To end a qi-giving session, remove your hands slowly at the end of an exhalation, when you have run out of breath.

Now that the mother has relaxed herself and stimulated her child by qi, it is an ideal time for the parent to introduce himself to the child by means of qi.

Have the mother lie on her back on the side of the bed. Bring a chair over close enough that both of your hands fit comfortably over the area above the pubic bone. Send qi to the fetus in the same way the mother did. It is not necessary to think her thoughts as you send qi. In fact, it is preferable to have your own thoughts that express your personality and wishes. This difference between mother and parent will be communicated by qi.

When the parent is the qi-giver, the mother should try to align her breathing with that of the parent and think positive thoughts such as the examples given above. You may want to synchronize your breaths by beginning together on the count of three, and then end the qi-giving session in the same way. (One-two-three, deep inhale, then exhale slowly.)

The breathing and positive thought-directed qi will induce a feeling of serenity and tranquility within the mother. The parent will also have to relax in order to send qi successfully. If, prior to giving qi, the parent has difficulty relaxing, he should lie facedown, and the mother should place her palms gently over his spine as in the exercise given in "You Relax Your Receiver," page 47. As she sends qi, she should include her child in the process by means of her thoughts.

"C'mon, Bun, let's send tranquil qi into ____."

"Bun and I are helping you to relax."

Within a minute, you will feel the muscles of the back relax, and then the spine itself will "loosen up," as if breathing a sigh of relief. The parent can now begin giving qi.

Remember: just as the health of newborns varies, so, too, does the health of fetuses. If the fetus is naturally weak, the qi you give will strengthen it, but not greatly. On the other hand, a healthy fetus will be greatly strengthened, her environment will be improved, and the subsequent months of pregnancy will become easier than they would be without qi treatments.

The baby usually will not rise within the mother until the second trimester. The baby may begin to rise as early as the eighth or ninth week, having a very slow ascent. The baby will rise considerably in the second trimester, as will be explained in that section. Should the baby begin to rise during the second half of the first trimester, she will probably not go far, only one or two inches.

The fetus will rise on the left side, just above the pubic bone.

Thus, toward the end of the first trimester (about the eleventh week), when giving qi, imagine that you are cupping the back of the baby's head in the palm of your hand. The baby will be about two and a half inches long (6.25 centimeters) and will look like, well, a little baby with fingernails, toenails, and eyelids. The baby's main organs are already in place.

Visualize the back of the baby's head, and send qi directly into it. By doing this, you stimulate the hypothalamus and thereby facilitate organ growth and development.

Talk to the baby. It will help with your transmission of qi.

"Turn your head to me, Bun."

"Show me that back of your head, Bun."

QI FOR MOTHER: STANDARD TREATMENT
FOR THE FIRST TRIMESTER

Qi for the fetus can be provided by either mother, parent, or both. Only the parent, however, can provide qi for the mother in order to guide her body in the healthy direction it wishes to go.

Since the moment of conception, the mother's body has been working toward two goals: (1) sustaining the child until it becomes capable of sustaining itself *ex utero* and (2) getting it out into the world.

Your body does not want to hold on to the child any longer than it has to. And why should it? So, for each of the 273 or so days your body is holding the child, it is moving toward a condition in which it can easily expel it and return to "normal."

Your body is going to change in terms of balance as your pregnancy progresses. This is perfectly natural. The fetus will grow in size, and you will have to grow proportionately to sustain it. The fetus will also change location during the three trimesters, and your body will try to correct any weight imbalance so that you can walk comfortably and avoid lower backache. Your spine will be under constant pressure, literally and figuratively, to modify its alignment in order to cope with the changes, and this is why flexibility is the key to a successful pregnancy.

The lumbar vertebrae are central to the processes of pregnancy and childbirth, in particular, the third lumbar vertebra (L3). The importance of keeping L3 strong and flexible cannot be overstated. L3 is responsible for maintaining the flexibility and integrity of the pelvis. During pregnancy, the strength and resilience of the five lumbar vertebrae are related to the strength and resilience of the seven cervical vertebrae.

We will therefore begin our standard qi treatment for the mother with the cervical vertebrae.

Cervical Vertebrae

The mother can be seated, lying on her stomach, or lying on her side. The first and second cervical vertebrae (C1 and C2) are located inside the skull. The parent's right hand should be placed at the base of the skull, and qi directed slightly upward.

When you have done this for two minutes, remove your hand (on an exhalation) and place it on the back of the neck, covering the remaining five cervical vertebrae. The last vertebra (C7) usually protrudes when the mother bows her head as if praying.

This makes it easy to find. After a couple of minutes of receiving qi, the mother should feel her neck relaxing. Continue giving qi for another minute, and then slowly remove your hand.

Lumbar Vertebrae

Place your hand on the base of the mother's spine, and send qi into it. L3 is located directly behind the navel. L2 is an inch above L3, and L1 is an inch above that. L4 is an inch below L3, and L5 is an inch below that (see "A Handy Guide to the Spine" on page 212).

Unless the mother is very tall, you should be able to cover all five lumbar vertebrae with your right hand. While you are sending qi with that hand, place your left hand on the mother's left shoulder. This creates a feeling of balance within the mother, and has a calming effect. It is not necessary to give qi with the left hand, but it does no harm, either.

Give qi to all five lumbar vertebrae with your right hand for three minutes. Remove your hand, and then place the heart of your hand on L3. Pressing gently, put qi directly into L3 for one minute. Remove both hands on your final exhalation.

The Face

The next treatment is to keep the ankles and pelvis flexible and aligned in order to alleviate or eliminate pregnancy rhinitis (sinus problems). It will also minimize or eliminate the headaches that many women experience on the sides of the head between the eyes and the temples.

The mother should lie on her back. The parent should sit or stand behind the mother, whichever is more comfortable, and place his thumbs on her face along the sides of the bridge of her nose. His other fingers can rest lightly on the sides of her head (see Figure 5.1).

Send qi through your thumbs into the face, and imagine that the qi is moving through the face, down the neck, along the sides of the body past the pelvis, and down the sides of the legs to the ankles. Continue giving qi for two minutes.

The mother can treat herself using qi. She can lie or sit upright, place her index or middle fingers alongside the bridge of her nose, and send her own qi through them, (see Figure 5.2). Or she can apply a hot compress or washcloth to the same points.

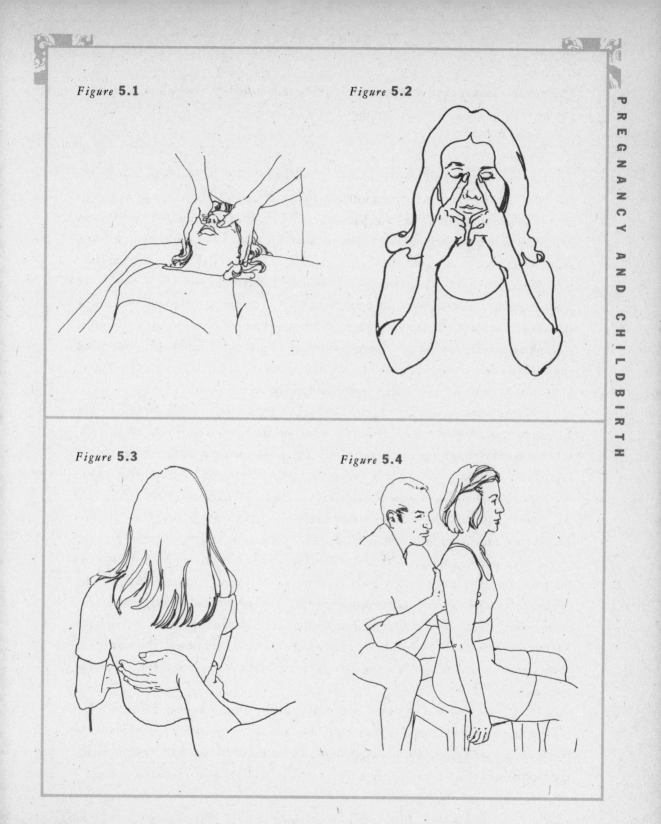

Figure 5.1

Figure 5.2

Figure 5.3

Figure 5.4

Using a compress is good, but it is not as effective as using qi, especially the qi of the parent.

Body Cleansing

The next three treatments are related to body cleansing. The human body is in a constant state of cleansing: we sweat; excrete; and produce tears, mucus, and earwax as various means of ridding our bodies of toxins and unwanted chemicals. Keeping her cleansing system functioning at peak performance is vital to the mother's health and sense of well-being. And, of course, the cleansing process is vital to keeping the child in a clean environment and promoting its own cleansing functions.

The kidneys are an important part of the body's cleansing system. Their healthy functioning is essential to keeping the fetus clean and the mother healthy. The mother can help herself by drinking more water than usual during pregnancy. This stimulates the kidneys. In cold weather, warm or hot water is recommended. However, it is up to the parent to provide qi in order to keep the kidneys in top form.

The kidneys can be reached from the back. They are located on either side of the spinal column, between the middle of the waist and the bottom end of the rib cage. To find them easily, place your forefingers on your navel, then move them in a straight line around your waist to your back. With the mother sitting or lying on her stomach, place each hand over a kidney and send qi into both for three minutes (see Figure 5.3)

Next, place the heart of your hand over T11, and send qi into it for a minute. This vertebra regulates kidney function, and it is important to keep it flexible.

The parotid (salivary) glands are also related to kidney function. Standing behind the mother (who is either seated or lying on her back), begin sending qi into Head Points Number 4. After a minute of this, cup your hands lightly around her neck, and send qi into the straight vertical line running from beneath the earlobe to the base of the neck for two minutes. (The parotid glands do not reach the base of the neck, but giving qi along the entire line both stimulates the glands and relaxes the neck muscles.)

Many women develop stiff neck and/or shoulders in the first trimester. The cause is usually tension in Head Points Number 4 (salivary glands). Thus, giving qi to the parotid glands reduces upper-body tension as well as stimulates the body's cleansing mechanism.

The lymph glands are also critical to the mother's cleansing mechanism. The mother should be seated. Sit behind her and place your hands, thumbs pointing to yourself, under her armpits. Raise her shoulders ever so slightly, and send qi into her armpits for one minute using the crescent part of your hand that touches the mother's body (see Figure 5.4).

During this procedure, the mother must be completely relaxed. It is up to the parent to hold the weight of her arms. The mother should not raise her arms or shoulders, nor should she attempt to "help" in any way. If the parent keeps his elbows tucked against his body, he will hardly feel the weight of the mother's arms.

The Waist

Finally, we wish to keep the mother's pelvis flexible and her sacrum in alignment with the lumbar vertebrae. Still sitting behind the mother, cup your hands around her waist directly under the rib cage so that the palms of your hands fit snugly over the sides of her waist. Send qi into the waist with both palms for a minute. Following this, you may gently gather the flesh of the waist in your fingers, and pinch ever so lightly three times.

From the time of conception until the moment of delivery, the mother should receive qi in her **cervical vertebrae, lumbar vertebrae, along the sides of the bridge of the nose, kidneys, parotid glands, lymph glands, and waist.**

Once you have a routine or regimen going, each session should not last more than fifteen or twenty minutes. Add to this about ten minutes for stimulating and communicating with the fetus directly, and the entire program comes to no more than thirty minutes per session.

Ideally, the mother should have daily treatments. However, three sessions a week are adequate.

WALK, WALK, WALK!

Cancel your gym membership and walk!

I will say it again: do not confuse fitness with health. Bearing a child does not require the ability to bench-press two hundred pounds. Nor is there any reason whatsoever to think that working out in a gym during pregnancy will speed up the return of your pre-pregnant figure. The program outlined in this chapter will restore your figure to its original state as quickly as your body is capable of managing. To believe that working out now will prepare you for childbirth or provide *postpartum* benefits is wishful thinking.

Consider this: You do not want to add any more physical stress or tension to your body, particularly the repetitive kind. Lifting and pushing and stretching will not help your body find the *integrity of balance* it seeks. Walking will.

Regular walking is the best exercise for a pregnant woman, and a wonderful way to do *in utero* child-rearing.

The woman should walk alone. This is because, rather than going out for a pleasant stroll with someone else, she has set aside special time to exercise with her child. This produces a psychological state that results in a strong flow of qi to the fetus.

Walking daily at a scheduled time "for the child" is a woman's natural means of sending qi to her child. Her qi will be concentrated on her child, particularly if she mentally or verbally keeps the child posted on what she is seeing on her walk.

"Oh, look, Bun, the Jacksons bought a new car."

"The roses are beautiful and fragrant. Can you smell them?"

"There's a nip in the air, do you feel it? It's getting on to autumn."

Nor can a gym provide the next benefit of walking. Walking accustoms the mother to dealing with a new center of gravity. Your balance will change, and walking will be a natural adjustment to that change. Walking regularly will keep you balanced properly and prevent falls. It will impart flexibility to the pelvis, sacrum, and ankles.

When you walk with your child, the two of you are a Mutual Aid Society. The child receives healthy, vigorous doses of qi and parental care, and the mother has her body balanced naturally.

Finally, walking will keep your stomach muscles firm without being hard or tight. You will not swell unnecessarily. A big belly is no indication of fetal growth. It is more important to have a firm, resilient belly. Your baby will not be harmed if you do not expand to blimp size.

MORNING SICKNESS

Morning sickness, or nausea, is said to affect from 60 to 85 percent of pregnant women. The numbers here are so imprecise as to render them almost irrelevant. The point is that more than half of all pregnant women experience some degree of morning sickness. The condition usually does not extend past the first trimester.

The human body is always in a state of cleansing itself. It is cleaning and cleansing in so many ways that the function may rightly be called an obsession.

The body releases its toxins through vomit, sweat, phlegm, saliva, tears, mucus, earwax, and, of course, urine and stool. Apart from isolated incidents, such as eating tainted food, receiving anesthesia, or falling ill, a woman's body never purges itself of toxins more than when she is pregnant. This is not only healthy; it is a welcome condition.

She is aided in this cleansing by her fetus who seeks to protect herself from toxins against which the mother already has an immunity. One source of such toxins is edible plants, all of which, to a greater or lesser degree, produce toxins. Postpartum humans have a detoxification system to protect themselves against these toxins. However, the fetus is sensitive and susceptible to even a small amount remaining in the mother's body. The fetus will try to reduce its exposure to toxins and will fight to reject any toxicity it encounters.

Tests have shown that toxins in potatoes cause neural malformations in animal fetuses. From this, it is conjectured that Ireland's rate of congenital neural defects, such as spina bifida, the world's highest, is due to overindulgence in potatoes. I am not suggesting that mothers swear off potatoes or products containing potatoes. I encourage them to eat a balanced diet without overindulging in any one thing.

The fetus develops its organs during the first trimester. It is therefore not surprising that at this important stage, the fetus should be sensitive to toxins. Nor is it surprising that the fetus, once stable, should be able to cope with toxins. This helps explain why morning sickness rarely persists past the first trimester.

Morning sickness performs a cleansing function. It may be purging your blood of toxins. It may be your child purging your blood of toxins. It may be a natural means of adjusting your body to the metabolic changes arising from pregnancy. A moderate to severe case of morning sickness may indicate that your body is overdue for a cleansing. By this I mean that your body needed a cleansing but, for any number of reasons (including stress), did not get around to it. Pregnancy initiated the cleansing process, and this process has manifested itself as morning sickness.

Therefore, though it may be unpleasant and uncomfortable, morning sickness is actually performing a useful function.

It is possible to accelerate the function of morning sickness in order to pass through it quickly.

TREATING MORNING SICKNESS

The Urinary Tract

The urinary tract needs to be stimulated. The procedure for this is described earlier, on pages 86–87. However, in the case of 90 percent of pregnant women, it is the right inner thigh that needs qi treatment. The long ligament on the inside of the right thigh will probably be tight and may even be slightly painful when touched or prodded. Send qi into the ligament for two minutes. Doing so will stimulate the cleansing mechanism of the urinary tract, and you will be aiding the morning sickness in performing its duty.

Liver

The parent should give the mother qi to the liver with his whole hand twice a day, first thing in the morning and about two hours before bed.

Diet

Instead of three meals a day, the mother should eat six to eight meals of small portions and various foodstuffs. **Eat only one type of food at each meal.** This will help relieve morning sickness and is useful in tracking down and identifying a nausea-inducing food. Carry snack foods with you, and eat as soon as you feel hungry.

Have a warm, nondairy drink about an hour before bed each night.

Having said this much about morning sickness, I will turn to the phenomenon of severe, ongoing, unrelenting morning sickness.

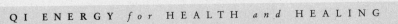

The best answer to give a woman who comes asking why she is having this truly dreadful experience is to say neither you nor anyone else on Earth knows.

Speaking from my own experience, two very plausible reasons may be given.

The first is "bad blood." Some women are simply unhappy being pregnant. Whether the pregnancy itself is unwelcome, or the parent is uncooperative, or the mother is constantly nervous and uneasy, or she is short- or bad-tempered . . . whatever the cause, the effect of this psychological state results in the production of toxins that the body tries to expel through morning sickness.

When the mother is "angry" with someone (including the fetus) or with her physical condition, in short, when she is "a bundle of nerves," her body tries to protect the fetus from "bad blood." The fetus herself, in self-defense, will cause or exacerbate the morning sickness as she tries to ward off the toxicity of the mother's personality.

In this case, morning sickness cannot be treated as one would treat a physical ailment. If you wish to use qi, it should be applied in large doses to Head Point Number 5, C2, and the entire spine in order to relax the mother and calm her head.

The second possible cause of severe ongoing morning sickness is trouble with the L5 vertebra. If the mother is aware of pain or discomfort in L5, or if you can feel that the L5 is sunken or depressed, you should give daily qi to that vertebra. The mother can be lying prone or seated. Place the heart of your right hand over her L5, and send qi into it for five minutes. You may also perform the treatment for L5/sacral pain given on page 105.

I have found that a combination of head/body relaxation qi and qi given directly to L5 produces positive results within ten days to two weeks. The persistent morning sickness does not necessarily vanish, but its severity is greatly reduced in most cases.

The Second Trimester

THE FUN TRIMESTER

If conception was the first milestone, you have now reached the second milestone. The third milestone is birth. The most worrisome trimester is behind you. You are now squarely in the least worrisome trimester. You can really relax and have fun.

Now is a wonderful time to begin thinking about names. Even if you plan to learn your child's sex prior to birth, you can still have fun writing down and crossing out boys' and girls' names at this point. What is important is to have a pleasurable, shared activity centered on your child.

This sort of pleasurable mental activity on behalf of your child directs your qi to her, and keeps her healthy and active. This is naturally true for the mother who is carrying the child, but it also stimulates the affectionate and generous qi of the parent. Transmitting qi becomes more of a pleasure as the "reality" of the child grows more substantial.

The mother will begin to show pretty soon, and she can think about buying maternity clothes. For goodness sake, do not let pregnancy derail or degrade your sense of vanity. Buy stylish, but also buy with a long-term view in mind, meaning a dress that will look good in the fifth month, but will also serve you well in the eighth month. Stores catering to pregnant women provide pillows to simulate your future expansion.

Think that pregnancy is making you more attractive. Go out and have fun shopping.

SEX

This is a great trimester to have sex.

It is safe and healthy to have sex from the moment of conception to the moment labor begins. In fact, in cases where the due date has passed without birth, intercourse may induce labor.

However, there are psychological and physical reasons why people avoid intercourse in the first and third trimesters.

Some fear losing the child in the first trimester. It is, after all, the time when miscarriages occur, and many couples prefer to abstain rather than "jeopardize" their precious fetus.

In the third trimester, the mother is "great with child." Now we arrive at a question of aesthetics. Many men find pregnant women extremely attractive and erotic; just as many men find them unattractive, even intimidating. The mother herself may, by the eighth month, find the child so heavy within her that she loses her sexual desire.

This leaves the second trimester. The pregnancy has taken, and the couple is confident that sex will not dislodge the child. The woman, though showing, is not showing to the point of aesthetic contention. Nor is the baby large enough to cause her physical discomfort. If we consider the second trimester to be the fun trimester, then this is certainly the optimum time to enjoy yourselves sexually.

Desire does not stop with conception, and consummation need not. And as you count the time to due date, remember that you will not be having *postpartum* sex for a pretty long time, especially if a C-section is performed.

MOTHER TAKES STOCK OF HER CONDITION

Let's take stock of your condition for a moment.

It is around the thirteenth week. Either alone or together with the parent, you have been giving qi to the back of the baby's head (occiput) for about two weeks. (At least you are imagining the occiput, or consciously directing your qi to it.) This stimulates the hypothalamus, which creates the stem cells that will become the baby's organs. The baby is now fully formed and recognizably a "person." Giving qi to the baby's occiput stimulates the growth and strengthening of the entire organism.

The baby now knows the qi of both mother and parent, and responds when given qi. The response may be a buzz, a tingling, a vibration, an emission of soothing warmth or refreshing coolness. Frequently, the baby will come to the heart of the hand, which is the source of the qi it is receiving.

Your child moves around the area of the pubic bone from right to left and back again. The baby will come if you call her with qi. Place your right palm over either the left or right side of the mother's lower abdomen just above the pubic bone. Now call your child aloud or mentally.

"Come, Bun, come to my hand. Come to the qi. It feels good, doesn't it? You love the sensation, don't you? Now come and have fun in your qi bath."

Or words to that effect.

If you have been giving your child qi since the first trimester, she will come.

If you are still unable to locate the child with qi, or if you do not feel your child's movement toward the qi emanating from your hand(s), keep sending qi anyway. The baby will soon rise within the mother, and you will then find her easily. She has been, and will continue, enjoying qi.

Your baby should be receiving qi at least five minutes daily. The more qi the better. Ideally, the mother and parent should each give ten minutes of qi to the child every day.

HOW IS THE MOTHER DOING?

She probably had a case of the "dropsies" for a short time from about the eleventh or twelfth week. Her body's balance is changing; the child has grown quickly and is preparing to rise within her. As she adjusts to the physical changes, changes in perception and tactile sensitivity are natural. Her body will naturally accommodate those changes, and she will no longer drop things. In the meantime, let someone else handle the fine china and stemware.

From the eleventh or twelfth week, it is possible that the mother will experience any or all of the following: sinus trouble, including stuffed nasal passages (so-called pregnancy rhinitis), sacral pain, and stiff ankles. Your nasal condition indicates that the pregnancy has well and truly taken; sacral pain and stiff ankles are indications that your pelvis is shifting to accommodate your pregnancy. Therefore, as in the case of morning sickness, consider that these discomforts are temporary and are signs of health.

If you have been following the regimen outlined in the first trimester, these troubles will be light and will not linger.

In order to alleviate the above discomforts, it is important to give qi to the sides of the bridge of the nose at this time, as explained on page 138. If this cannot be done, warm to hot compresses should be applied three times daily, for three minutes at a time.

Any morning sickness or nausea should be tapering off or completely gone by now. If mild nausea remains, this will gradually disappear. Should medium to severe nausea persist, it is time to begin giving qi to L5, and stimulating the urinary tract as directed on pages 86–87.

The mother's tastes in food and drink should have returned to "normal" by now. For mothers who experienced medium to severe morning sickness, taste may run to something stronger and spicier than usual. Mothers tend to stick to bland, even tasteless foods in the hope of avoiding nausea, and once this fear has passed, the palate craves something dramatic.

The mother is eating for two in terms of health; she is not yet eating for two in terms of quantity.

It is not necessary to eat more than usual or more than is comfortable thinking that your child will go to bed hungry unless you do so. At this point, you still have enough body fat to supply the child with plenty of food.

TALK, TALK, TALK!

Bun is without any life experience, and has absolutely no knowledge of how you live and function in the world.

Well, from the beginning of the second trimester, you are going to enlighten him. He may be ignorant, but he's not incurious. Bun is very curious and needs you to fill him in on what is going on.

It is time to begin talking out loud to your child in a natural, unaffected way, telling him all about what you are doing. If you care to, you may even tell your child why you are doing it.

"I'm going out now. I'm taking the car and going to the market to buy food, and you're coming with me. We're going shopping together. I have a list of fruits, meats, vegetables, and dairy products that I am going to shop for, and then we'll come home and put them all away neatly. We need to eat in order to live, though sometimes I think your Uncle Al lives in order to eat."

Your child needs to be informed of what is going on around her. You can begin your child's toilet training from this time.

"Mommy's going to the toilet. This is how it's done. She pulls down her pants, and sits down. It's very comfortable. This is what you'll be doing one of these days, by age two, I hope. Anyway, then Mommy . . ."

Of course, playing harmonious and melodious music to your child in the womb is a fine thing to do. For some reason—perhaps because he revealed his genius from infancy—Mozart is favored by the expecting public, and some claim his music will even improve fetal intelligence.

Sure, why not?

It is, to me, more important to talk and talk to the child. Your child will respond to the tone and timbre of your voice. You are not talking away from your child, as you do when you have conversations. You are including your child in your world through language and feeling.

Bonding with your child as you educate her through spoken words will, of course, enhance the efficacy of qi communication. Remember: qi is intention. Bonding and education go hand in hand. The child knows when you are speaking, and she knows when you are not speaking to her. The worst thing you can do is "ignore" her.

If you have been walking daily as advised earlier, but speaking to the child mentally, it is now time to give your words voice as you stroll along together. If you have not begun setting aside time to walk with your child, get into the habit now, before she rises within you in a couple of weeks.

And as you walk together, talk together.

QI FOR MOTHER: STANDARD TREATMENT FOR THE SECOND TRIMESTER

Sorry, Mom, the preferential treatment could not last forever.

At the beginning of your pregnancy, your body experienced so many changes that you were given priority of qi treatment. Even if your child received only two minutes of qi daily, you were sure to get at least ten to fifteen minutes of daily treatment.

Now, you and your child will be running neck and neck, neither of you having priority. And when the child rises, priority changes from you to him.

Qi treatment for mother in the second trimester can be given with her lying on her back.

Keep giving daily qi to both sides of the bridge of the mother's nose. Do this straight through the pregnancy, and even after the mother has given birth.

Achilles Tendons

Go to the mother's feet, and raise them from the heel. Cradle the Achilles tendon of each leg with your hands, the heart of the hand directly over the tendon (see Figure 4.35, page 123). Your thumbs and forefingers should be touching her ankles.

Send qi into the tendons with your entire hand(s). Imagine the qi traveling up her legs, up along the sides of her body, over her shoulders, through her neck, and up into her head from where it exits into space.

Do this for at least four minutes daily. It will relax her head and ankles. In the case where the mother's ankles are painful or tight, give qi for five to six minutes.

Feet and Ankles

It is also important for the mother to keep her ankles and feet warm. Wear socks around the house. Do not go barefoot unless you have underfloor heating and the floor itself is warm.

I also recommend soaking the feet to the top of the ankles twice a day in warm/hot water. The water should be between 100°F and 105°F (body temperature is between 98°F and 99°F). Fill a foot basin or other receptacle with warm/hot water, and place both of your feet in the basin so that the water covers your ankles. **Leave your feet in the water for three minutes.**

When you remove your feet, they will be nice and red. Pat them dry, and put on thick socks to keep the heat in. Not only will this keep your ankles flexible and alleviate stiffness, it also will provide a pleasant jolt or stimulus to your nervous system.

The Head

Have the mother raise her head slightly, and place your hands, palms up, under the head to cradle the sides (see Figure 5.5). Send qi into the head through your palms. Do this for two minutes. Remove your hands slowly on an exhalation.

Give qi to Head Points Number 2 for two minutes a day.

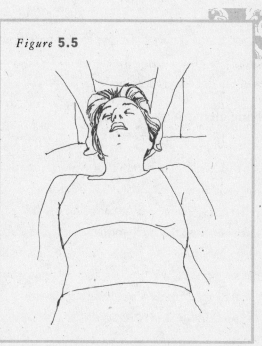

Figure **5.5**

L4 and Sacrum

You should no longer have any trouble locating L4. This is just as easily done from the front as from behind.

Slide your hand, palm up, under the mother's back so that L4 rests on the heart of your hand. Send qi into L4 for two minutes.

If the mother's sacrum is stiff or painful, slide your hand down from L4 so that it covers her sacrum, and send qi into it for two minutes.

The above covers the standard procedure for qi treatment for the mother during the second trimester. There is nothing at all wrong with carrying on the regimen of the first trimester if time allows, **especially body cleansing through the function of the kidneys.** To keep a steady flow of water circulation, therefore, make sure you drink about eight glasses a day.

LO! THE BABY RISES!

It is week fifteen, approximately day 107. The mother awakes to feel something has changed. She is not sure quite what is different, but that something is different is certain.

Now, many mothers will not feel any difference. They will have no idea where their baby is until he kicks. There are all sorts of photos and illustrations and anecdotes of the mother bowled over with joy when, after about eighteen weeks, her child gives her a swift kick, and his existence becomes "real" to her.

But you have been qi-playing with your child, talking with him, monitoring his progress, giving him qi baths, and so on, and you are very aware of his whereabouts, and much more so his "reality." So you place your hands just over and above the pubic bone and call him, but he does not come. In fact, he does not even seem to be around. You do not get a response from him as you usually do.

Your child has moved.

He has avoided the intestines on your right side, and moved upward into your lower abdominal area on the left side.

To be as precise as possible, the baby is now three fingers' width down from the left side of your navel, and is there to stay for a while.

In about two weeks, you will feel a slight, round bulge at this area. This is the back of the baby's head, which is now well formed. This is the spot you have been sending qi to since the eleventh week, and this is the spot you will continue to send qi to throughout this trimester.

From the end of the seventeenth or eighteenth week, the baby will flutter her arms and legs when she receives qi to the occiput. At first, this is an involuntary movement. Her movements will feel jerky. The reflex activity of her extrapyramidal motor system is at work. As qi continues passing into her, her movements will seem to become more conscious and voluntary. You will feel a change in her movements between the first minute of sending qi and the third. If you continue giving qi for more than five minutes, she should calm down and emit a strong, steady flow of qi into your hand.

By the end of this trimester, you and your child will have created a qi routine that entertains and satisfies you both.

By the twenty-first week, the baby will begin to hiccup. The application of qi may set this off, or it may occur spontaneously. Continued application of qi will cause the hiccups to subside.

By the time a week has passed after the baby rises, the mother will notice that her balance, her walking, and her posture have become slightly different. If she and/or the parent have been monitoring her body, they will notice that her hips have opened slightly. The pelvis is now preparing to open to full expansion for birth. This does not mean that full expansion will occur anytime soon—that won't happen until the day of the birth. However, the body is gauging its own flexibility and moving in the direction of full expansion. By all means, keep giving qi to the L4 vertebra.

And keep walking! Keep up your daily routine of walking with your child and talking to her.

EDUCATION AND DISCIPLINE

If you did not know before, you now know exactly where your child lives.

But not, alas, where he hangs out.

He shifts and moves and squiggles all through the mother, and so is not always easy to find. Sometimes he makes the mother uncomfortable by sticking his foot or fist down into her crotch, and she doesn't know how to get him out.

Now is the time to use qi as a disciplinary and educational tool.

If the baby is not "at home," place the heart of your hand three fingers' width down from the left side of the mother's navel, and call him.

"Come to the qi, Bun."

"This is _____. You know me and my qi. Come over for a chat."

"This is your mother talking to you. Pull your toes out of my crotch and swim over here to my hand. I need you to help me with this."

It is very important to get your child involved in her own birth, which you can do with qi. As you put qi into her, you should explain to her that what you are doing and what she is experiencing are all just part of getting born. You will explain her role in the process (she is the star), and that you will not ask anything of her that she is incapable of doing. You have to give her a time frame, an itinerary if you like, and a good idea of how she is to behave and when.

"Right now you're free to roam around Mommy's belly, and you'll be able to do this for another couple of months. But about two months before birth, we'll ask you to settle down and remain in a certain position. Don't worry, we'll tell you what position long in advance. And after you do that, we'll tell you exactly what you have to do to get born."

Your child will want to cooperate as a partner, because she is grateful for all that you do for her. You may say, "How do you know this?" The answer is that qi babies are extremely cooperative and eager to please before, during, and after birth. (Actually, I believe that all babies are cooperative; they have just not been educated into the *means* of cooperation in the womb. They would cooperate if they knew how. . . .)

Qi babies are different from non-qi babies in four ways. The first is that you can make requests and demands of a qi baby that you cannot with a "traditional" infant. (The other three differences are apparent after birth. Qi babies are remarkably wrinkle-free and have a gloss and sheen to their skin. Qi babies show an alertness and curiosity at the moment of birth. This lasts only about twenty seconds, but it is real. Qi babies have a low center of gravity, and so feel that they have more "bottom weight" when you hold them.)

If you really need him to sleep that extra hour on Tuesday, he will. If you need her to poop before Grandma arrives, she will. If you need him quiet on board an airplane, sucking both on take off and landing, he will. All you have to do is ask. That is what I mean by cooperation.

Qi babies are not angels upon whom you can place limitless demands and responsibilities, but when it comes to cooperating on important points, they will do all they can to oblige.

Now is the time to give your child a sense of responsibility and opportunities to cooperate. You do this by talking aloud to your child as you send her qi.

"Bun, I can't do this without you. You've been a champ so far, and I want your help with the rest of the pregnancy. Listen to what I ask of you, and do whatever you can. For the time being, I just need you to get your elbow out of here."

"Honey, don't be restless right now. Mommy's tired and needs her nap. We'll play in an hour or so."

You will be surprised how your qi child will accede to your requests and demands.

The parent is also very important in instilling a sense of responsibility and discipline in the child. It is fun to spend time with the mother and child, your hand on her belly, giving your child a sense of belonging to the family as you stimulate her with qi.

"Bun, Mommy loves you and has been taking great care of you. I love you, too, and take good care of you and Mommy. We need you to come when you're called, because we like to know where you are. So when you feel me or Mommy calling to you, come over as soon as you can."

"You're a funny kid, you know that? So I'm going to give you some funny qi. I'm going to tickle you with qi. It tickles Mommy, too, and you can feel her laughing with you. Go on, laugh together."

If *in utero* education and discipline as described above strike you as harebrained or frivolous, well and good. At the very worst, it is a harmless exercise in bonding that will help the mother and parent pass time together in an agreeable way.

However, I have no doubt that you will find that "lines of communication" develop between you and your child and that by the time the child is born, all three of you will have a well-defined and accurate idea of one another's character and personality. There will be no surprises when you meet face-to-face. And what is more, your child will be disciplined and susceptible to your wishes outside the womb.

What is neither harebrained nor frivolous is the intention of training your child to participate at his own birth. You have to be able to get your child to do what you want him to do *in utero,* so that he will respond to your directions if guidance becomes necessary.

More specifically, it is important to be able to tell if the child is settling down and positioning himself correctly for birth. If he has not, you should be able to turn the child within the womb by having him follow your qi as you trace a line or circle on the mother's abdomen. You will need to monitor your child's position from the beginning of the third trimester, which is why it is vital to begin training your child to respond to you now.

From the end of this trimester, approximately week twenty-five, you should start putting your child to sleep at your bedtime. (This training can begin as early as week twenty-three.) The mother more than ever needs a deep, restful sleep, which she will not get if the baby is active within her. Moreover, this is the time to start inculcating sleep patterns and habits. If your child is on a regimen by the time of her birth, you will be spared a lot of sleepless nights over the first three years of her life.

The mother needs to be relaxed before bed. This can be done by qi relaxation techniques, warm drinks, or both. Many women find that warm milk is relaxing, but makes them feel bloated or gives them gas at this time. Warm low-fat or nonfat milk is tasteless and unsatisfying. Anything with sugar, such as cocoa, should not be taken.

Warm water with a touch of lemon juice is good. There are many varieties of herbal tea that are tasty and whose aroma induces relaxation.

Next, the mother will lie on her back. Her belly is large by now. Both she and the parent probably know where the baby's head is. At this stage, the baby is turning, if not already turned, head down.

Place your *left* hand on the back of the baby's head, and your *right* hand somewhere (anywhere) else on the baby's body. Give qi with both hands.

As you send qi into the baby, talk to her, and tell her that it's bedtime.

"We're all going to bed now, Bun. You're not missing anything by sleeping. Get comfortable. Suck your thumb and settle down for the night. We will wake you up in the morning and play again. I promise."

Or words to that effect.

You will find that very soon your baby will cooperate and sleep through the night.

A prenatal sleep regimen is an extremely valuable gift that the mother and parent can give themselves. And Bun will appreciate it, too.

Finally, you should be able to train your child to come to your qi when called in order to penetrate the cervix with his head when labor begins. This is a great aid in accelerating and measuring dilation, and gets the birth off to a promising start. Both this and changing your child's position will be dealt with in the third trimester section.

Though training the child with qi is done for a serious purpose, that does not mean training should be undertaken with gravity and high seriousness. The best education is a playful one. Mother and/or parent, alone or together, can induce the child to play "follow the qi" from the time the baby rises. Once you have located your child (and I recommend starting from her "home") and have sent qi into the back of her head, it is time to get her moving.

Move your hand in different patterns over your abdomen, and see if the child follows. Up and down, side to side, diagonally, in a zigzag. Get her to turn somersaults by very slowly describing a circle on your belly. The main thing is to have her enjoy your qi, and to respond to it as asked. And while she is enjoying herself, tell her how much she means to you, and what you expect of her and why.

Remember: educating and disciplining your child are different from talking to her.

Chatting and gossiping or simply conversing with your child should be done without the direct application of qi. The mother's qi will naturally stimulate the child as she talks to her. The child will be grateful to be included in the mother's activities of daily life.

CASE HISTORY

The mother will start to show from about the twentieth week. Any time after this is a good time to ask the baby to tell you its sex.

Place your right hand on the baby's occiput, and while sending qi into it, say, "I want you to tell me if you are a boy or a girl. If you are a girl, buzz my hand with qi once. If you are a boy, give me two buzzes."

Then finish giving qi on an exhalation, relax your hand, and wait. You should have an answer within thirty seconds. If you do not, or if you are unsure of the reply, ask again.

Our child said boldly and clearly that he was a boy on two occasions, once in the fifth month, and once in the eighth month. No one else agreed with him. The Japanese fortune-teller predicted a girl. Some physicians, based on the rate of heartbeat, predicted a girl. (Boys are supposed to have a slower heartbeat than girls. Our baby's heartbeat was a slow and steady 130 beats per minute when monitored by qi at home. When he went to the OB/GYN, his rate would climb to 140 to 145 beats per minute. It might have been Therese's influence, but then again, it might not. In any case, the elevated heartbeat had people thinking he was a girl.)

The Mexican *bruja,* or sorceress, had no doubt we were having a girl. The yentas in the supermarket said it was obvious we were having a girl from the way Therese was carrying. A clairvoyant saw our child in a dream—a lovely tow-headed girl.

And finally, we had a pricey Beverly Hills gynecologist perform an ultrasound scan two weeks prior to due date. He looked exactly like Liberace and had much the same manner. I expected him to place a candelabrum instead of a scanner on Therese's belly. He concluded we were having a girl. (This dismayed us, since we had specifically asked him not to tell us the sex.)

Therese gave birth to a boy.

Our child had told each of us twice he was a boy. It must have driven him crazy to be called Miranda for the last month of his *in utero* life, and to hear his mother and her friends talk about how they planned to dress "her."

I have asked seventeen fetuses to tell me their sex. Thirteen answered correctly.

The Third Trimester

LET'S GET THIS SHOW ON THE ROAD

At the beginning of the third trimester, the baby weighs about two pounds. By the time you deliver in thirteen weeks, the baby will weigh anywhere from six and a half to upward of eight pounds. The baby will grow about seven inches in length during this time, from about fifteen inches to about twenty-one or twenty-two inches.

The seventh month begins with a bang. It is a time of excitement for the mother. The baby, who has been moving around inside of you, will begin to turn. Bun should be head down by the thirty-first week. As the baby turns and begins to settle into the pelvis, there may be some vaginal discharge, but this is nothing to worry about.

At the thirty-fourth or thirty-fifth week, the baby stops taking iron from the mother, and the mother's iron count rises. This coincides with a feeling of heaviness. It is from this point that many mothers begin counting the days until the due date. They get bored and uncomfortable, and begin to wonder why this reproductive process takes so damn long!

This month, the eighth, is perhaps the most difficult of the pregnancy, particularly if the baby is inactive. The mother's boredom keeps her from being active, which leads to tightness in the pelvis, which in turn leads to an even greater sense of boredom. It is now that pregnant women report feeling as though they are carrying a bowling ball inside of them.

Do not stop walking, and if you have access to a pool, try to swim or walk through the water daily. This activity will keep you strong and flexible, and if you talk to the child as you walk, it will take your mind off the bowling ball. Go out and shop for baby clothes. It is refreshing and reassuring to look at clothes for newborns, and realize that your child is actually going to arrive as a tiny thing. The small size of the garments is a healthy counterweight to the size of the baby as it now feels inside you.

The baby gains weight rapidly. As the baby descends into the pelvis, the mother's visual acuity begins to decline. Objects do not appear as sharp and focused as usual. (Vision will return to normal after birth when the pelvis regains its alignment.)

Varicose veins or spider veins may appear. The baby is putting pressure on your diaphragm, so breathing may be a little difficult. As the baby drops and finally settles into the pelvis at the end of the eighth month, breathing becomes easier, and the lower back does not feel as much strain as before.

The ninth month becomes one of anticipation and activity as the due date approaches and the mother and parent share a sense of the reality of birth.

This anticipation is not always of the welcome kind. It is all too easy to become uneasy or anxious about the birth itself. This unwelcome anticipation puts tension into the pelvis, which is quite the opposite of what is best for an easy childbirth. The birth is not the mother's responsibility, and she should feel no "performance anxiety."

The pelvis will open and close dramatically. This is a natural movement. The pelvis will adjust itself nicely in time for the birth. It will be tight or constricted only if there is a mental effort to force it open before its time. You cannot move the pelvis by psyching yourself up or by willing it to open. Your attempt will block the body's natural adaptation to the condition of giving birth.

At this point, rather than think of birthing a baby, think of having provided a sheltered haven to a living thing for nine months, and that living thing is going to come out on its own.

"Conventional wisdom" holds that older women have more difficulty giving birth. This is true only if they allow themselves to be badgered into "trying" to give birth before the body is ready. Age is not a factor—an "older" woman has just as much flexibility and resilience as a "younger" woman. It may be truer to say that older women will have easier births for they tend to be more relaxed, sedate, and inclined to let Nature work slowly.

Nor is a previous C-section a hindrance to a vaginal birth. Relaxation and an awareness that the baby will actively strive to be born and that you will be cooperating with it rather than forcing it out will contribute to a successful birth.

Finally, do not spend time or effort concentrating on the due date. The date is merely a signpost, not a divine decree. I have read that only 5 percent of all births occur on the due date. If you allow a certain date to become a preoccupation, you will be putting stress into your body. Remember, each day that the baby remains inside the womb is another day of healthy growth and development.

QI FOR MOTHER: STANDARD TREATMENT
FOR THE THIRD TRIMESTER

Carry on with the same regimen of treatments as hitherto, with particular attention given to L4, the urinary tract, the sides of the bridge of the nose, and the Achilles tendons. If/when the mother's vision becomes fuzzy, you can apply qi directly to the eyes. The mother lies on her back and closes her eyes. Place your index or middle fingers lightly on the eyes, and give qi for two minutes daily.

L3

From the eighth month, it is important to keep L3 flexible. L3 is the command post issuing orders for getting the pelvis to open and close before and after birth. If L3 is twisted, pelvic movement will be inhibited, and the birth may well be difficult. Further, a twisted L3 at the time of giving birth will lead to lower back pain in the near future.

It is especially important to monitor L3 in women who have experienced a miscarriage.

The mother may be sitting or lying on her side. The parent places his thumbs alongside L3 and, pressing firmly but gently, puts qi in for three minutes daily. Then place an index or middle finger directly on L3 and give qi for two minutes.

L1

L1 is also very important to childbirth. In cases where the due date is long past, L1 should be checked. It will probably be protruding and need large doses of qi.

From the beginning of the ninth month, giving daily qi to L1 will accelerate the mother's *postpartum* recovery process.

EDUCATION AND DISCIPLINE

If you think of birth as a graduation from womb to world, then Bun needs to be informed all about the graduation ceremony and her part in it.

When the baby descends into the pelvis, the back of her head is just above the pubic bone. It is easy to find and fits nicely into the palm of the right hand. Give Bun qi every day for at least ten minutes, and talk about life on the outside world as often as you can—tell her about the color of her room, about her sleeping arrangements, about the toys you have for her, and about the adoring grandparents and others who will bill and coo over her.

From the beginning of the ninth month, it is time to educate Bun into the birth process.

"Mommy's womb is going to move. It is going to try and push you out. Then Mommy's hips will open wide, and you will be able to get your head out. We want you to help us when the action begins. We want you to bounce and bounce against the cervix and push yourself out. We really need you to cooperate, and we know you will because you love us and want to help." Or words to that effect.

From the ninth month, the parent can place his hand on the back of the baby's head and encourage him to bounce. There is not much room for movement, but the baby can move his head down into the cervix as a rehearsal for the graduation ceremony. Thus, when it comes time to be born, the parent can root the baby on with his hand on the back of the head and sending qi: "C'mon, Bun, bounce down, bounce down for all you're worth. Let's get this show on the road."

Qi babies are cooperative and will do their utmost to please their parents. If you have been communicating with your baby by qi at least from the thirteenth or fourteenth week, you will be amazed at how eager your baby is to please you and win your approval.

Childbirth

It is not a "fact" that giving birth is painful and difficult. Only about one in a hundred pregnancies involves difficulty, and it is better to concentrate on the successful ninety-nine than on that one. Most women hardly remember what it was like to give birth, though most will remember their pregnancies. The mother should be directed to think of the joys, past and future, that her pregnancy and childbirth provide, and intend to have an easy, sensual birth when the process begins. On no account should the mother be told to be "brave" or to use willpower to fight against pain. As soon as the idea of pain is introduced, tension arises in the mind and body, and this tension impedes the natural flow of the mother's qi from producing an easy childbirth.

The mother gives birth in ebb tide, and the baby is born in flood tide (see page 113). When the mother goes into ebb tide within two weeks of the due date, you may confidently expect the birth within a few days. When the signs of ebb tide become pronounced in the mother, the baby will be born within two days.

Do not lie in bed waiting for the due date and time. In fact, the pelvis opens about eight hours prior to childbirth. The opening of the cervix follows this. At this point, most mothers think that childbirth is imminent, and they grow tense. This leads to forcing the birth, which leads to pain. In fact, there may be as long as eight to ten more hours of waiting from this moment.

When labor begins, walk a lot at home. When step turns into shuffle and the knees feel weak, it is time to go to the hospital or to call the midwife. The belly will feel warm to hot and will be buzzing with qi at the point where the belly curves down at the pubic bone. In cases where the parent has been instructed in how to check for dilation of the cervix, this is the time to check.

If you are having a normal pregnancy and childbirth, there will be a feeling of pressure or an ache around S2. When this ache ceases and the feeling moves south to S4, the baby is on her way.

The main point is to be relaxed. Do not lie in bed waiting for something to happen. Keep walking until something does happen.

GIVING BIRTH

Most couples will have attended birthing classes, and the parent will have been taught how to coach the mother in breathing during childbirth. The parent will also have been instructed to encourage the mother to push the child out.

Qi looks at things the other way.

The mother should not tense with each wave of pain, but should exhale powerfully in order to relax. As she exhales, she should be sending the exhalation breath to her pelvis and imagining that both hips are spreading to maximum width. She should leave the birth up to the child.

Once the baby's head crests, the parent should have his hand somewhere on the mother's body. If she is supine, then it is natural to place the hands on her belly. If she is on all fours, the parent can place his hand over her L3–L4. In either case, the parent should be encouraging the child to come out.

"We need you to cooperate now. Come on and get yourself born. Come out of Mommy and into the world where we can all see you."

Or words to that effect.

The point is to remove the "onus of childbirth" from the mother, and let the child be responsible for her own debut into the world.

After Giving Birth

Congratulations! You have a healthy, well-loved child. The child is, of course, unable to care for herself, and needs your attention. However, to be an effective mother and a good source of nourishment, you should take care of yourself and be taken care of by the parent.

After the birth, you should not put any weight on your pelvis for at least two hours. If possible, stay off your feet for at least five hours. Remember, birth requires the pelvis to be at maximum expansion. Staying in bed gives the pelvis time to realign and begin its movement toward closure.

The mother does not truly lactate until the third or fourth day after giving birth. What is initially produced is a fluid called colostrum. Even if you do not intend to breast-feed, it is very important to have your newborn take as much colostrum as he can. This thin, yellowish fluid is rich in protein and calories. It also contains a great amount of antibodies and lymphocytes.

The *postpartum* health of the breasts and lactation are directly related to pelvic movement. Richer milk in one breast indicates that the left and right sides of the pelvis are not closing at the same rate. The breast of the side that is closing more slowly will have the richer milk. Your baby will prefer one breast to the other, and this indicates the quality of the milk. If the mother does not intend to nurse, it is good to pump milk or massage the breasts in order to promote flexibility of the pelvis.

The pelvis does not close all at once, but gradually, one side a little bit at a time until the end of the first week. If, for example, you step out of bed within an hour after giving birth, you will be putting weight on one side of the pelvis (the leg that first touches the floor and bears the weight). This will interrupt or stop the closing of the pelvis on that side. The milk in the breast on that side will be rich, and there will be the possibility of breast infections in the future. The baby will not want to suck from the other breast.

After the first *postpartum* week, the hips will begin to close simultaneously. At this time, it helps to close the hips by walking an hour or two each day. This puts natural tension back in the pelvis and aids in equal closure on both sides. If both hips close equally, both breasts will have equally rich milk. The nursing infant will not prefer one to the other, and the mother will not end up with one breast looking like a tortilla after weaning her child.

So, following childbirth, the pelvis contracts, then opens, then contracts, then opens, all the while tending toward closure. It is this pelvic movement that results in discharge (blood) from the womb. Light discharge tapering off about the end of the third week indicates healthy pelvic closure. If a heavy discharge continues past four weeks, it is an indication that closure is not progressing in a healthy way. The entire process should finish by the end of the sixth week.

The closing of the pelvis also supports the spine. If the spine does not return to its former alignment, lower back pain will ensue within a year.

During the first three weeks after giving birth, the mother should take things slow and easy. If possible, the parent or someone else should do housework and prepare meals. It takes a full six weeks for the pelvis to return to its prebirth condition. Ideally, the new mother will have nothing heavier to lift or carry than her newborn during that time frame. Resting for six weeks following childbirth will restore the mother to her original level of energy, ensure she has a good supply of milk, and restore her body's shape to its pre-pregnant condition. When the pelvis returns to its original state, the mother's eyesight will also return to normal.

The pelvis may be stimulated to close by giving qi to L3, L4, and L5. Further, following birth, the parent should give qi to the mother's ovaries. This will help remove any debris still left in the womb and will accelerate pelvic closure. Do not put anything cold on the ovaries. They need warmth. Giving daily qi to the ovaries will restore the pelvis to optimum flexibility.

Lila was thirty-two years old, and came to see me ten weeks after giving birth to her first child. Her complaint was that her right breast was three times the size of the left, and so full of milk that she felt it would explode. Her left breast, on the other hand, produced almost no milk. Her baby would not suck the left breast no matter how appealing she tried to make it, even going so far as to dab a bit of syrup on her left nipple.

I naturally asked her about how soon she had put weight on her pelvis after giving birth. "Immediately," she replied.

She had given birth squatting in her bathtub, and stood up and climbed out of the tub as soon as the baby had popped out. She had put all of her weight on her right leg. Her right pelvis had frozen at maximum expansion the moment she did this, and though the left pelvis was closing nicely, her right side still had not moved since the birth.

I gave qi to her right ovary, her L3 and L4, and to the right side of the bridge of her nose. I told her to put a hot compress on the right side of the bridge of her nose twice a day, to soak her right foot up to the top of the ankles, and to walk at a comfortable pace for thirty minutes a day.

After a week, her right pelvis was closing. As it did, her left breast began producing more milk. After two weeks, her baby drank from both breasts equally. The right breast was no longer swollen, and the left breast had grown so that both were the same size.

CHAPTER 6

The Very Young and the Very Old

The First Years

It is true that we are helpless at birth. Just sitting up is a milestone. It takes a year before we can walk clumsily. Our organs require years to develop fully. Many people's minds never develop fully, as evidenced by the intellectual quality of daytime television shows. We have no language at birth, and we are unable to hold a musical instrument, much less play it. All of this development takes time.

On the other hand, we are born with astonishing flexibility, both mental and physical. An infant can suck his toes. An adult who can suck his toes earns a living as a yoga master or a circus contortionist. We acquire our native language in a remarkably short time span from birth, and the more we age, the longer it takes us to learn a foreign language. By the time we reach middle age, learning a new language, even one as "logical" as Esperanto (the international language), becomes a chore.

167

Children absorb the novelties of their environment and digest them like nutrients. They display insatiable curiosity and delight in having mind and body stimulated. To many an adult, "there is nothing new under the sun," and they become remarkably incurious and jaded.

The same holds true for qi. Thanks to her natural flexibility, a child is far more susceptible to qi treatment than an adult. Of the forty minutes spent on a single qi treatment, thirty minutes go just to relaxing the adult so that his body is flexible enough to change through qi. Young children, on the other hand, change almost instantly by means of qi, and a treatment takes little more than five to ten minutes.

Moreover, young children really feel the qi as it enters them and moves within them. It is a delight to watch children receive qi; they look as if they are receiving one of life's great treats. Place your hand on an infant's belly and put qi in. The child will erupt in burps, belches, hiccups, farts, and sneezes, and have a thoroughly good time. A child who has not been feeding well will vomit up some undigested food, and then begin to eat like a trencherman.

Until he entered first grade and was given homework, my son's final words each night were, "Work on me, Papa." He found it very soothing and reassuring to receive qi before bed. A bit of qi to his lower spine, and he was in dreamland. Once the demands of school increased, we had to make "dates" for qi, and other means were employed to put him to sleep.

Children are so sensitive to qi that, unless the child has a serious physical problem, no finesse or technical expertise is required to maintain the child's health. As a concerned and loving parent, you can put your hands anywhere you like on your child's body, and be assured that the qi will go where it has to go and do what it has to do.

From the age of four (three if the child is precocious), children who regularly receive qi will begin to want to give it. The joy of giving qi back and forth between parent and child is unique among the pleasures of parenthood. In terms of vitality and effect, a child's qi is no different from an adult's; Junior's qi will keep Senior healthy.

If your child went through the qi program outlined in the previous chapter, he will (1) be glossy and shiny, (2) have relatively few wrinkles, (3) show a curiosity and awareness from the first, and (4) feel substantial when held. Most babies feel light, as if the weight is in the head; qi babies feel solid and balanced from the bottom (backside).

There is one last characteristic that will become apparent later. Generally, boys tend to speak later than girls, and children who are placed in day care soon after birth speak sooner than those who are kept at home. Qi boys who are kept at home tend to speak quite late. Their energy is going into their physical and physiological development, and so they retain their "baby characteristics" longer than other children, and their speech is delayed. This does not mean language does not exist within the child; it is just not demonstrated as early as in the case of non-qi boys. The same goes for qi girls. Their speech will not develop as quickly as that of their counterparts. All qi kids begin speaking from the same age as non-qi kids, it is just that their "verbal skills" are not as advanced until the age of four. From the age of five, qi kids will start talking a blue streak.

Just because the child lacks the verbal skills of his peers does not mean that his language comprehension is deficient. Quite the opposite. He understands perfectly everything you say from the same age as other children.

Just as a stray animal matures faster than a well-kept house pet, so a well-loved, well-raised child given a healthy diet of qi retains his childish qualities longer than other children. There is no hurry for your child to become "adult." Your child will catch up gradually. In the meantime, enjoy her "babyness."

Because they retain their "baby characteristics" longer than non-qi kids, qi kids maintain their playfulness and curiosity longer than non-qi kids. Furthermore, I have never met a qi kid who suffered from attention deficit disorder or required Ritalin in order to cope with schoolwork. Qi kids stay focused from an early age. They are also eager to please in order to be rewarded with parental approval. This makes them manageable and easy to educate.

Newborns

In the past, babies were born at home. Today, most are born in hospitals, though there is a trend to returning to the home as a birthplace. When babies are born at home, it is possible for the mother to lie with the baby after the birth. The baby has just left a balmy 99°F for what must seem like a cold climate. If the baby can lie on the 99°F mother, it will soon adjust to the new temperature. Further, the mother can perform her first maternal responsibility, cleansing her child of meconium.

In a hospital birth, the baby is taken to an "incubator" to stay nice and toasty until mother and child are reunited. In this case, it is up to the parent to cleanse the child of meconium.

Meconium is the first feces of a newborn. The child is stuffed with it. Meconium tends to be greenish-black, and has the consistency of tar. Don't even bother to wash the towels you catch it in; just discard them. The first meconium should come out during the first twenty-four hours after birth and, under normal circumstances, finish after about three days.

In the world of qi, the faster the meconium is released, the healthier the newborn becomes. Relieving the newborn of meconium directly after birth aids in preventing skin diseases, allergies, and childhood diseases, and generally strengthens the child. It also provides the first *postpartum* bond between mother/parent and child.

The newborn can go without food for twenty-four hours. There is no hurry to feed him. When the meconium is evacuated, the newborn's appetite is stimulated and he will suckle in quantity.

Sending qi to the newborn's liver will induce the evacuation of meconium.

As in the case of an adult, the newborn's liver is located directly beneath the rib cage on the right side. It is very small. The tip of the index or middle finger will cover it. If the baby is with the mother, she should put a towel under the infant, place her fingertip over the liver, and send qi in for five to ten minutes. If the newborn has been removed to an incubator, the parent can do the same procedure there. By giving qi, meconium will begin to be released within ten minutes, and the entire process should end by the second day.

Meconium is odorless, but very sticky. Do not touch it if you can help it.

You can stimulate the newborn to suckle by the application of qi to Head Point Number 5. Hold the baby in the "football" position so that the palm of your hand naturally cradles the back of the head. Send qi into the back of the head, and the baby will respond with a sucking reflex. Now that the child is born, it is possible to use the left hand as well as the right hand for sending qi.

If the child is thus stimulated to suck by qi, and if the meconium is being released, you should get the baby to "latch on" and suckle within two hours after birth.

Remember: the mother is not yet lactating. The colostrum she is producing is vital for strengthening the newborn's immune system.

Babies need a lot of water. Put lukewarm water in a baby bottle and add an approved sweetener and just a trace of lemon juice. This will taste like mother's milk. You can give the baby water for a minute before giving her the breast. Feeding the baby water from a bottle, and pumping milk and feeding it to the baby from a bottle at nighttime will accustom the child to drinking from a bottle. Babies without bottle experience tend to reject a bottle later, and so transition from breast to bottle is difficult. You can successfully wean your baby by starting him on a bottle soon after birth.

CASE HISTORY

Harry's wife delivered by C-section, and the newborn was taken from her immediately and placed under a heat lamp inside a plastic "incubator." Harry went to the nursery together with the newborn. When the nurses left, he stealthily placed the tip of his middle finger over Josh's liver, and sent qi. The heat from Harry's arm set off an alarm, and he had to remove his hand quickly and stick it in his pocket, and whistle nonchalantly.

When the nurses returned to their station, Harry removed the heat sensor from Josh's body, and began giving qi to the liver again. After about six minutes, the meconium began to appear. Some passing nurses stared suspiciously at Harry, who once again removed his finger and replaced the heat sensor. He would have like another couple of minutes to give qi, but the "dark deed" had been done.

Two maternity ward nurses came into the nursery and saw the meconium coming out. Cleaning meconium is a chore, and neither was happy. They shooed Harry out of the nursery and cleaned up Josh, who by this time had released about 40 percent of his store.

An hour later, Sarah took Josh in her arms, and sent qi into Head Point Number 5 as she listened to the maternity nurse lecture her on the difficulties of latching on, and how not to be disappointed should Josh show no interest in her breast. Josh abruptly ended the lecture by latching on and sucking noisily.

Infants, Toddlers, and Young Children

RELAXATION AND SLEEP

Human beings experience the world through their feet long before they use their hands to get to know their environment. Infants lie on their backs and wave their legs in the air as if they were the antennae of an insect. It is through the legs, the Achilles tendons in particular, that infants, toddlers, and young children can be relaxed and put to sleep.

Whatever sensations the infant is experiencing are sent into the brain where they become part of the "hard wiring." It takes about three years for the hard wiring to be completed, and those first three years are a time of intense mental and physical growth and development. The child's brain is literally buzzing as she seeks to make sense of the stimuli. Without comprehension of the structure and order that define patterns of stimuli, we would be overwhelmed by our environment. Much of an infant's crying is simply a heartfelt response to a stimulus/sensation that she cannot mentally comprehend, and that includes hunger and tiredness.

By means of qi, it is possible to stimulate your infant to eat, and then relax him to be tranquil and sleep. If you are prepared to spend a little time creating a pattern of behavior, your child will soon fall into the structure of the pattern and cooperate with you. This will eliminate sleepless nights and many tears, both yours and theirs.

With the child on his back, hold his heels in your hands so that the Achilles tendons are resting on the hearts of your hands. One leg will seem "colder" than the other, and the qi will not flow into it as smoothly as into the warmer leg. Send qi into the tendons just as you would in the case of giving qi to an adult. When the cold leg warms to the same degree as the other leg, the child will relax and show signs of sleep.

It is also possible to give qi to the Achilles tendons while holding the child. Recline in a comfortable seat and hold the child to your chest, heels facing out. If the child will lie still, place the hearts of your hands over the tendons and give qi. If the child will not at first cooperate, have the parent give qi while the mother holds the child to her chest.

Qi to the Achilles tendons will relax a child up to the age of six. It is from age six or seven that the pulmonary system verges on completing its development, and so children from age seven require the same relaxation procedure as in the case of adults.

CASE HISTORY

Josh "got with the program" from the day he came home from the hospital. Sarah stimulated his Head Point Number 5 to suckle every two to three hours, and then gave qi to his Achilles tendons to make him tranquil and sleepy.

Sarah pumped milk and put it in the fridge so that Harry could feed Josh during the night. At nighttime, Josh was fed at four-hour intervals by the same process, qi first to the head, then to the heels.

Both Sarah and Harry gave qi to Josh's liver after each feeding. This stimulated his natural cleansing system.

Josh fell into this structured behavior from the end of the second week. He was fed and had his diaper changed twice during each night. As a result, neither parent suffered from loss of sleep. Because of his familiarity with a bottle, Josh was easily weaned off the breast in his seventh month.

YOUNG LUNGS AND EAR INFECTIONS

A child enters the world with his lungs a clean slate. Suddenly, he encounters pollen, dust, the scent of cheap aftershave, the smell of food, and so on, all of which force themselves upon his unsuspecting lungs. No wonder children sneeze and cough a lot. And no wonder they cry a lot. There is nothing like a good cry to cleanse and invigorate the pulmonary system. "Out with the bad air, in with the good." It is a natural form of *kiryū* for the lungs and good for the child, no matter how awful it may be for bystanders.

Air enters us via the nose and mouth, and then passes through the throat into the lungs. The ears are also related to the nose and throat, and so infectious organisms entering the lungs can also enter the ears. This is one of the causes of ear infections in children.

There is no protection against infectious organisms other than to strengthen the body's immune system and cleansing system. That is why it is important to give qi to a child's liver daily or at least twice weekly from birth. That is why it is important to give qi to the child's T1–4 three times a week if possible.

Horizontally placing two adult fingers at the base of a baby's neck will cover the first four thoracic vertebrae. These vertebrae are responsible for pulmonary function, and so keeping them flexible promotes the development of the lungs. In children over four years old who have asthma, the first three thoracic vertebrae will be tight, and T4 will usually be protruding or prominent. When a child has asthma, check for a groove between Head Point Numbers 3 and 5. If a groove is present, do the procedure given on pages 82–83. If no groove is present, treat the asthma as you would anxiety or a sleep disorder.

T1–4 should be given qi regularly until the child's lungs are fully developed at about age seven.

Ear infections also occur when the child's first assertions of independence are thwarted. Children seek to assert themselves from an early age, and are already testing the bounds of their autonomy from age two. "No" being the most common word in the new parents' vocabulary, the child's assertions have many opportunities to be thwarted. The child responds by throwing a temper tantrum. It is important to nip the conditions for a tantrum in the bud at these times by diverting the child's attention away from his assertion and the parent's rejection of it. A lengthy tantrum or a series of tantrums can lead to an ear infection.

When the child's desire for autonomy is thwarted, he becomes extremely frustrated, and the qi within him gets blocked in the abdomen, causing the organs to tense and even twist. This impedes the body's natural cleansing functions, particularly the urinary function. You will find that the child does not urinate as often and as easily when he has an ear infection. While he is napping or sleeping at night, the urine will be released, either as bed-wetting or waking him so that he has to go to the toilet.

To promote inner-ear healing, it is important to give the same treatment as you would for the urinary tract in adults.

CASE HISTORY

Josh had only one ear infection during his life, and that occurred when he was two and a half years old. Harry and Sarah took him to a birthday party at a pizzeria geared to children. Josh was quickly caught up in an ecstasy of screaming, eating, running around, and playing games.

After two hours, it was time to go home, but Josh vehemently refused his parents' requests to say good-bye. When they lost patience and demanded that he leave at once, he threw the only temper tantrum of his life. He had to be physically carried out of the restaurant, kicking and screaming. It was not until he had been strapped into his car seat and the restaurant was out of sight that Josh calmed down and became his usual self. Harry and Sarah thought he felt feverish, but that was only to be expected after that prolonged and violent outburst.

The next day, Josh woke up holding his hand over his right ear, and complained of pain. The ear did indeed feel feverish, and Harry and Sarah suspected an ear infection. They kept him home from preschool. He urinated only twice during the day and wet his bed at naptime. Sarah gave him hourly doses of qi directly to the ear, to his liver, and to the inside of his left thigh. By the evening he felt better, and by the next morning, he was able to go to school.

To return to the lungs: Most children's pulmonary system begins developing quickly between ages three and six. The lungs are in a state of flux. Ages four and five are a particularly important stage for the development of the bronchial passage, lungs, and affiliated body parts, such as the nose and throat. This involves a lot of cleansing, which takes the form of mucus. Cleansing mucus tends to be thick and yellow. Runny noses in children of this age are a normal reaction to excitement and other stimuli to the system. The mucus is frequently accompanied by a cough or a bout of coughing. This developmental process can be accelerated by giving qi directly to the lungs. Sitting behind the child, place your hands on the child's back just where the rib cage ends, and send in qi with both hands. After a minute, the area beneath your hands will feel warm. After another minute, the child's breathing will deepen. That is the signal for you to stop giving qi. If the child coughs, lower your hands further along his back and continue giving qi for a minute.

Next, hold the child's right upper arm and give qi as explained on pages 49–50. This will relax his upper back.

Dry coughing at night in a child between ages three and six is the body's own spontaneous attempt to relax the T1–4 vertebrae. During the day when the child is active, the four vertebrae will move and stay flexible. It is at night that the body can align itself naturally. Coughing maintains these four vertebrae in alignment and thereby promotes pulmonary development. If you feel the four vertebrae before bedtime, and then after the child coughs in her sleep, you will notice a difference in quality of flexibility.

THE PELVIS

The modern parent is eager to have her child participate in "physical enrichment" programs from an early age. This means "kidnastics," kiddie yoga, kiddie soccer, kiddie martial arts, and any number of other physical and competitive activities. Added to this, the child is riding her tricycle from age two or three, and graduating to a bigger bike by age four. All of this impact puts considerable stress on the pelvis and lower limbs. In the case of girls, especially girls doing gymnastics, this stress can lead to problems with pelvic movement later in life, and these problems can affect fertility and childbirth.

From the age of four, a child's pelvis and lower body develop quickly. It is important to maintain the strength and flexibility of the pelvis during this time of development. The child can do this himself, or the parents can help with qi. Ideally, the child will do his part, and the parents will do theirs.

The child should be encouraged to bounce from one leg to the other, as if he is doing a dance, something like a sailor's hornpipe. Two hops on the left followed by two hops on the right followed by two hops on the left, and so on; this may be done to music. The child will enjoy the exercise and keep it up for a minute or so—all the time that is required if the exercise is done every day.

The parents can also help their child's pelvis. The child lies on his back, legs outstretched and slightly apart. The parent stands over the child.

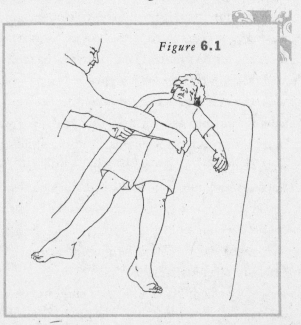

Figure **6.1**

With the fingertips of the right hand, tap firmly on the left hip six or seven times, and then press the fingers into the hip and give qi for a minute. Do the same thing to the right hip with the left hand (see Figure 6.1). Next, pull the child's little toes (pinkies) gently; stroke his legs starting from the knees and extending to the tips of the toes; massage his calves lightly; finally, place your hands over his ankles and put qi in for one minute.

Parents should give qi to the child's sacrum on a regular basis. Doing this will help keep the pelvis in alignment.

The Elderly

> *Wrinkled with black spots,*
> *Bent back, bald head, white beard,*
> *Trembling hands, wobbly legs,*
> *Teeth falling out, failing hearing, failing vision,*
> *Wearing a headscarf and glasses, walking with a cane,*
> *Fearful of death, lonely,*
> *Greedy, impatient, foolish, nosey,*
> *Annoying, and bossy,*
> *Praising one's children in the same old stories,*
> *Proud of one's health,*
> *Hated by everybody.*
>
> —ZEN MASTER SENGAI (1750–1837), "Afflictions of Old Age"

The image of the elderly has hardly changed today.

Sengai was a kind-hearted man, and his poem was meant as gentle irony. However, it is hard (especially for people who do not deal directly with the elderly) to realize that while much of what Sengai describes is true, much can be prevented, alleviated, or tended to.

The defining feature of aging is loss of flexibility. Eventually, this loss becomes so great that we return to the helplessness of the infant. We become dependent on the help and goodwill of others. This is not a welcome condition to someone who has been to some degree autonomous since age two, not to mention someone who has held positions of responsibility and managed to raise a family.

A decline in autonomy frequently leads to an alteration of the character of our qi; we become, as Sengai wrote, "greedy, impatient, foolish, nosey, annoying, and bossy." These are not attractive characteristics, yet they certainly provoke an immediate and powerful response, which is something that dependent elderly enjoy.

The physical loss of flexibility is apparent. Everything from vision to stamina to hearing to recuperative power declines. There is nothing anyone can do about this, no matter how many "anti-aging" products one devours. It is doubtful that the loss of flexibility can even be delayed or retarded. Diminishing flexibility is part of the human condition and has to be accommodated rather than mourned. New avenues that allow us to utilize what flexibility remains should be pursued. The growth and spread of senior centers is a recent phenomenon that provides new avenues and outlets to make the most of our reduced capacities.

On the other hand, within this physical decline, it is possible to fulfill our potential for health and flexibility by giving and receiving qi, and by doing *kiryū* on a regular basis. The phrase "within this physical decline" is of supreme importance here, because it defines the parameters of health. A program of qi is not going to rejuvenate an eighty-year-old body into a fifty-year-old body. It may improve eyesight, but it will not restore it to teenage levels. It will not bring back acute hearing. It will alleviate aches and pains, but it will not prevent them.

It will bring out the full potential for health and vigor available to *that* **eighty-year-old body.**

Loss of physical flexibility is frequently accompanied by a decline in mental and emotional flexibility. The person who was once grateful and cooperative for any and all help received now becomes cross-grained and bad tempered.

To put it another way: **What was once a flow of qi of cooperation becomes a cycle of resistance and conflict.**

The elderly person's behavior becomes an expression of that resistance. Cooperation seems like a further loss of autonomy, while resistance is felt to be an assertion of independence. A spirit of harmony and conviviality brings about a weakening of the qi, while argument and aspersion bring fire and strength back to the qi.

To digress for a moment in my allusion: The Japan Socialist Party (JSP) was, from the time of its inception, an opposition party. And oppose it did. . . . The JSP was a very skillful opposer, and its resistance to government policies and projects kept it lively and healthy. Suddenly, through a vagary of political fate, the JSP came to power in the mid-1990s and was in a position to enact policies of its own. The trouble was, it had none. It had become so used to opposing as a reflex response that it had never developed any creative or constructive vision. Once the party came to power and there was nothing left to oppose, it withered and died.

The same holds true for many of the elderly whose qi has altered through lack of flexibility of mind. These elderly people want to be harangued, pleaded with, and cajoled.

"If you don't get out of bed, you'll get bedsores and have to enter a nursing home. You have to get out of bed every day and do a little walking."

"You should let me cook for you. Eating ice cream three times a day is not a healthy diet."

"You can't insult your attendants like that. They'll quit and then where will you be? Good help is hard to find."

If you were to agree with everything the resisting elderly said, and let them have their way on every point, they would follow in the footsteps of the JSP, and wither away.

To many of the elderly, resistance is a natural form of *kiryū*. It keeps them sharp, alert, and vigorous. They are not seeking a confrontation that demands a "yes or no" resolution. To force a confrontation to a resolution would probably leave them at a great disadvantage from what they presently enjoy. What they are seeking is an on-going dialog that tests strength of will.

Thus, a refusal to change an unhealthy lifestyle, such as poor diet, or an indulgence in antisocial behavior, such as verbal abuse or smoking, is a natural form of *kiryū*. The elderly person actively seeks to provoke reactions that will force her to resist even more. She seems to be selfishly trying to get her own way. This is, to a certain extent, true. She is also stimulating her cleansing mechanism through resistance. Her physiology becomes energized. Moreover, resistance binds the caretaker or family member more closely to the elderly person, providing the elder with a sense of security.

"I can't just walk away from her and let her decline even more. After all, she is my mother, no matter how bad her behavior is."

This may seem perverse. After all, most people are willing and happy to care for their elderly loved ones. Honey attracts more flies than vinegar, and so harmony is a more powerful bonding agent than conflict. However, by resisting and provoking conflict, the elderly person feels that she has the upper hand in the bonding process; that it is she who writes the script that you willy-nilly follow, rather than vice versa. *She* becomes much more active and involved in the bonding process if you have to harangue her for fifteen minutes to take a walk, rather than were she to acquiesce and hop out of bed at your first suggestion of healthy behavior.

The closer the elderly come to death, and the more the idea of death intrudes upon their consciousness, the more they will resist and reject as a self-strengthening endeavor.

This is, to friends and family, tedious and irksome behavior. It is also an interesting phenomenon, vital to a true understanding and appreciation of the human organism, and how it seeks to make itself strong and healthy by any means available. The justness or unjustness of your advice and demands is not an issue with the elderly person. He will resist in the same way he will reflexively scratch an itch. And, as in the case of scratching an itch, it provides him with relief and satisfaction.

One way to bring an elder "out of himself" and get him to exercise his qi in a positive and harmonious way is to seek qi from him. The strength of qi does not decline with age, and the qi of a ninety year old is every bit as potent as that of a twenty year old.

The elderly often enjoy talking about health matters, especially the declining health of others. There is almost nothing that produces a glow of schadenfreude in the elderly like hearing a younger person complain about a health problem. Should you divert the elder from his attitude of resistance to one of assisting you and yours with your health problems by means of his giving you qi, you will be redirecting the thrust of his natural energy from rejection to generosity, and thus helping it enlarge.

Just have the elder place his hands on his grandchild, his great-grandchild, or any passing child you can lay your hands on, and tell him to direct the qi of wisdom and longevity into the child (or into you or your spouse). Breathe together with the elder. Synchronize your breaths and imagine a harmony of spirit. You will see that, as the elder gives qi, his shoulders drop, his abdomen relaxes, and his breath deepens. These are all healthy signs.

mn braces. Bless relaxes." Rather than the negative
ergy of providing what blessings you still can pro-
s caretakers.

of the elderly would say, "I don't want to give my
e my energy with him. Here, take five dollars from
l keep him happy."

preferred the qi of resistance to the qi of generos-

yert the resistant elder is to do *kiryū* together. The
hen under the influence of *kiryū* as younger people.
ngly. You can test this by placing your hand over
do *kiryū* together. You will find that the qi swirls
e elderly frequently yawn during *kiryū,* and may
doze off at the end of a session.

QI TREATMENTS FOR THE ELDERLY

Very few people enjoy their old age, especially extreme old age from eighty-five plus
years. I am told "Screw the Golden Years!" by almost every elder I meet, my own family members included. I will probably say it myself if I make it that far.

One of the phenomena arising from this lack of enjoyment is a tendency of qi to
collect in the heads of the elderly. Another is poor digestion.

Whether it is reminiscing about their youth, or reliving a pleasant event, or settling old scores in the mind, the elderly are very much absorbed by thoughts. If the
thought is of the nature of a pleasant reverie, it will relax the person. If, however, the
thought is repetitive and nagging, it will lead to erratic behavior.

Too much repetitive mental activity, especially of a bitter nature, will obstruct
sleep, circulation, and pulmonary function. When this occurs, appetite declines, and
so the overall level of energy suffers.

**Giving qi to the elderly should not be prolonged. It should be short and
intense.** A brief, intense burst of qi to an elder can fill the person with all that is
needed for the day. If the elder actually enjoys the feeling of receiving qi, then by all
means, place your hands anywhere that is comfortable to him, and send qi for as long
as he likes.

Stomach

It is good to slow the activity of the mind, relax the body, and have the qi collect at the stomach. It promotes mental relaxation, and improves appetite and digestion.

Have the elder lie on his back. When he is comfortable, the two of you take three slow breaths together. On the final exhalation, place your right hand just below his solar plexus and directly over his stomach. Send qi with your whole hand. Within a couple of minutes, you will feel the area beneath your hand grow very warm, and this warmth will spread across the entire abdomen. Continue sending qi until the elder's breathing is slow and steady, and then remove your hand slowly.

Lungs

As in the case of the very young, the very old need a lot of qi to their lungs.

With the elder on his back, sit behind him. Place your thumbs alongside the neck where it meets the shoulder. There will be a dimple or groove at this spot. Pressing gently but firmly, send qi directly into the dimples for a minute, and then release quickly.

You can also stand at the side of the elder and, placing your hands over his rib cage, send qi directly into the lungs.

Heart

The elder is still on his back. Standing to his right, place your left hand over his liver. Your right hand will go under his left armpit so that it is in line with his heart, located beneath the sternum (breastbone) (see Figure 6.2). The fingertips of your right hand will be touching the floor or table.

Send qi from your left hand to your right hand for thirty seconds. Then send qi from the right hand to the left. You will feel that the qi flows more powerfully in one direction than the other. Send qi for two minutes in the more powerful direction. If you do not feel any difference in strength, send from the liver to the heart.

The effect of this procedure is to strengthen the heart and improve circulation.

Do not give qi to the head of an elder who has suffered a stroke or head injury.

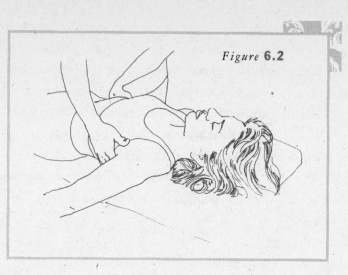

Figure **6.2**

CASE HISTORY

Samuel, aged eighty-five, was the very picture of an old curmudgeon. He had been a successful clothier and raised two children who produced a total of three grandchildren. Until his late seventies, he had been sweet-tempered and cooperative. His lower body had lost strength from about age eighty, and he relied on a walker or a wheelchair to get around. His personality changed when he began losing his powers of locomotion.

Now nothing pleased him. He was critical of everyone and everything. His family was frequently reduced to exasperation by his verbal abuse and lack of cooperation.

Samuel might have continued indefinitely in this pattern had his wife, Naomi, not been hit by a car in a supermarket parking lot. She sustained a serious, but not life-threatening injury to her head. When she came home from hospital, Samuel became her caretaker and teacher. She had lost a large chunk of her vocabulary and had no sense of taste.

He was not strong enough to look after her physical needs, but he made sure that the attendant was scrupulous in fulfilling his duties. He actively participated in every facet of his wife's care, including her diet.

Finally, he came to me to learn how to give qi in order to accelerate her healing.

Because of the nature of her injury, he could not give qi directly to her head. He worked on her stomach, heart, liver, and lower back, which had also been injured in the accident. He sat behind her while she watched TV, and sent qi into her lungs. As her recovery progressed, he could feel her qi flow more steadily, and this feeling energized him even more. His wife made a full recovery in less than a year. Her speech returned to normal, and food tasted as it always had, although she now had a craving for salt.

Samuel passed away three years later. He liked to call himself the Santa Claus of qi. He doled it out to friends and family, especially to his two new great-grandchildren. His family missed him very much.

CASE HISTORY

My Aikido instructor, Takeshi Watabe, is a model of successful aging, and part of the reason is his fondness for giving and receiving qi. Another part of the reason is that he became a teacher at the cusp of "old age," from age sixty, and remained eager to teach through his extreme old age. He is, at the time I write this, still teaching at age eighty-seven. As eager as he still is to teach, so there are students eager to learn from him, and a healthy give and take of energy is the highlight of his old age.

Mr. Watabe is a small man and could not compete in strength with an average-size man, especially an average-size American man. Added to this, he did not begin his study of Aikido until he was forty years old, by which time he was considerably past his physical prime. This meant that he had to rely on qi to become a proficient martial artist. As he put it, "Making the right move at the right time."

And so he trained his qi, his breath, and his sense of timing, so that strength and size became irrelevant to his understanding of Aikido. His technique was always fluid and flexible. It never fell into a pattern of "do such-and-such in so-and-so situation." His technique came from his personality and the refinement of his qi. It did not come from repetitive imitation of a martial art paradigm.

He did not spend forty-seven years practicing Aikido in order to become a hero or a warrior or to protect himself from attack. He practiced in order to develop his qi and to maintain his health. He enjoyed learning and he enjoyed teaching. He enjoyed the company of people who enjoyed exercising their qi. He avoided people who exercised only their strength. A proficiency with qi gave him the ability to "read" people and situations, and he rarely did not make the right move at the right time.

His qi was of its very nature and cultivation a constructive rather than a destructive qi; in other words, his was a healing qi. He maintained a mental and emotional flexibility long after his body lost its nimbleness. Still, his body responded remarkably quickly to qi treatment. He suffered an accident at age eighty-six that twisted his sacrum and pelvis, leaving him in great pain. It took only two short treatments to restore him to his original shape and health.

Thoreau in *Walden* tells the parable of the artist of Kouroo, who, "As he made no compromise with Time, Time kept out of his way, and only sighed at a distance because he could not overcome him." In the same way, Takeshi Watabe made no compromise with size and strength. Therefore, when he reached old age, he had neither size nor strength to lose. He refined his qi, which kept him vigorous, flexible, esteemed, and in harmony with his environment. The infirmities of old age only sighed at a distance because they could not overcome him.

CHAPTER 7

Sexuality

Sexual Energy

It has always seemed to me that, among all the animals of the world, only human beings have got sex down right.

In the first place, nonhumans are impelled to sex through dark evolutionary pathways. Male and female can spend the entire year ignoring each other when suddenly instinct kicks in and they go into heat. If it isn't *that* time of the year, there is no possibility of sex. They are slaves of biology. Their sexual energy arises, is quickly expended, and then subsides for another year or so. How unlike us, who can have sex three times a day every day of the year if we like. Or never have sex during our entire lifetime if we choose. Certainly, among animals, only humans have sexual energy throughout the year and maintain our sexual energy long after the possibility of reproduction has passed.

Only human teenagers are sexual slaves of biology, subject to their raging hormones.

Nonhumans have sex in order to reproduce. There are no secondary gains or ulterior motives. Humans do, too, but they also have sex in order to have fun, in order to make money, in order to learn state secrets, in order to commit blackmail, in order to acquire and wield influence, and for any number of other wholesome or unwholesome reasons. The motives for sexual activity are so diverse that they constitute one of the bases of world literature. Homer's gods were a sexually rowdy lot, and as for Anna Karenina . . .

Look at sexual behavior in the nonhuman world. It usually involves mayhem and may lead to murder or death. For most nonhumans, foreplay consists of two males going into combat to impregnate a female they hardly know. And when the contest is over and the loser is dead or maimed, and the winner staggers over to his prize, she usually puts up a fight or at least an argument against consummation. Sometimes she eats the male! There is a lot of wham and bam, but never even a "thank you, ma'am." Human sexual behavior is, by comparison, tame and mild.

Human males rarely if ever fight over a woman, especially Homo americanus, who prefers to litigate. True, there is the *crime passionel,* but this has to do with jealousy, and jealousy is usually an alloy with possessiveness as its primary constituent. Moreover, human beings have chosen to regulate their sexual behavior by religious injunction and instruction, legal restraints, social taboos, or any combination of the three. There is no "age of consent" or concept of chastity in the nonhuman world.

I suppose that jousting for a woman's favor was the last time human males clashed formally as a sexual rite; even then, the winner was assured only of receiving some sort of token from the female, not necessarily a sexual favor. Medieval romances would have us believe men fought each other with lance, sword, and shield in the hope of winning an embroidered handkerchief.

Nonhumans have very limited sexual tastes. They stick to their own kind and rely on heterosexual relationships with fertile partners as their object is pregnancy rather than anything else. Human beings combine an "anything goes" attitude with an if-it-feels-good-do-it rationale for their behavior. Human sexual taste includes same-sex relationships, fertile and infertile relationships, and incest. If the jokes and anecdotes found throughout the world's civilizations from ancient Roman times to the present about human dalliance with horses, donkeys, dogs, and sheep are any indication, human sexual taste is as broad as it is possible to be.

I imagine that the dildo preceded the invention of the wheel. There is no civilization that has not created gadgets and toys related to sex. Nonhumans lack devices and contrivances for expediting and enhancing the sexual experience. In fact, most nonhumans lack an interest in creating an ambience as an aid to sex. No soft lights, no music, no wine, no prenup agreement, no waterbed; just a patch of mud, some dusty grass, or a rock in the sun.

And where method is concerned, nonhumans are hopelessly mired in evolutionary tradition. No *Kama Sutra, Perfumed Garden,* or tantric scrolls for them. Whereas nonhumans are limited by evolution and nature, we humans are limited only by our imagination. In other words, our sexual energy is as much mental as physical. Here is where we, indeed, differ from the rest of the animal kingdom.

Our sexual energy is not confined to our genitals. It is also found in the ligaments of our bodies, in our chests, and in our heads. The mind/body unity is nowhere more apparent than in the simple activity of an assignation. We think about the meeting, count the moments until it is time to meet, our chest tightens, our muscles tense, and we conjure up our partner in our mind's eye. This diffuse energy unites in an explosive moment in our genitals in which supreme tension is followed by supreme relaxation. Then we make plans for the next meeting, and our bodies adapt and adjust to the pleasure of anticipation.

Sexuality is not necessarily related to sexual performance or the act of sex. The mind/body unity allows us a multiplicity of channels for our sexuality.

Sexuality is related to the amount of energy we put toward sex in one or more of its various forms.

We think of sex or sex-related things from an early age. We continue to think of sex into our seventies and even into our eighties. Thinking of sex creates a flow of energy between our minds and our genitals. **This flow of sexual energy creates our uniquely human attributes, beginning with desire.** Desire for fame; desire for possessions; desire for food; an adventurous spirit; creativity; religious faith; an active, forward-looking personality—these human characteristics are all products of the flow of sexual energy. This energy, unless it is impeded, flows within us until the moment of death.

As long as the flow of sexual energy is unimpeded—as long as we have a healthy sexuality—we create, desire, demand, accept, hope, and act in a positive and vigorous way. We see the world as a place where the sun shines, flowers bloom, the sky is blue, and the wind blows. When the flow of sexual energy is impeded—when the urge for sex in any of its forms departs from us—the world becomes a gray, unfriendly place.

We become timid, indecisive, and gradually grow inward until we have retreated into our minds, ending up with little else but unproductive repetitive thoughts. We grow rigid and harden. When this occurs, we begin to decline and deteriorate as human beings. The sad thing about this condition is that, thanks to modern conveniences and social amenities, we can continue in this state of deterioration for years and years without dying. We are neither dead nor waiting for death. We are living in a colorless, indeed a lifeless, world, in which sounds are muted and colors have lost their vibrancy. Our desires deteriorate. We never know satisfaction because our desires are so paltry. Life is bleak.

Sex complicates our lives, even if the sex thought or act is solitary. I do not mean by this that sex leads us into temptation and delivers us unto evil. I do not mean the complexities of human relations that are created through the act of sex. I mean that sex, in thought or deed, stimulates and energizes us. Sex invigorates us. Sexual energy inflames our desires and stimulates our creativity. For better or worse, the world becomes a vibrant, pulsing, noisy place that is not always congenial to us. Our fate as full-fledged human beings decrees that we maintain our energy, fulfill our individual potential for health, cope with and participate actively in this bustling, difficult world.

I was, of course, being facetious in my comparison of human and nonhuman sexual behavior. However, there was a core of seriousness behind the joking tone. Nonhumans are driven by instinct, and so sexual behavior is simple and "natural." Humans are driven by many different motives, and human sexual behavior usually deviates from the simple and "natural."

Camping is now an elaborate affair that requires lots of props and planning rather than just hunkering down in a cave after a day of hunting and gathering. It requires planning, transportation, and equipment that our primitive forebears would find laughable. In the same way, sexual behavior now requires planning, transportation, and equipment that our primitive forebears might have envied. Just think of the colossal "sex industry" that includes everything from magazines to gadgets to alcoholic beverages to lingerie catalogs. The intricacies of marketing sex reflect the complexities of our civilization and the distance our sexual behavior has departed from the simple and natural. People whose sexual energy would be channeled into nonsexual behavior—sculpting, writing, painting, marketing, mountain climbing—when the sexual urge declined, are now expected to perform sexually regardless, and sexual aids and medications are provided to effect that end.

To repeat what I wrote earlier: Sexual energy is not necessarily related to sexual performance or to the act of sex.

A loss of sexual desire or a decline in sexual performance does not necessarily reflect a loss of interest in life. A loss of interest in life is always reflected in a loss of sexual desire or declining performance.

A loss of sexual power does not mean that the individual's qi has waned. It may be redirected to other more interesting or satisfying channels. However, a loss of interest in life means a decline of sexual energy, and the flow of qi will be impeded throughout the body. People who experience a loss of interest in life become prematurely old. Their sexual energy dries up. I call the phenomenon "premature aging." Premature aging can occur any time in a person's life. In some men, it occurs as early as the thirties. It can also occur as late as the seventies or eighties.

Premature aging means that, though there is still plenty of life in the body, there is neither urge for, nor thought of, sex in any of its diverse forms. There is no invigorating tension in the chest, in the ligaments, or in the mind. Because of the mind/body union, the vitality of each declines. The mind loses its clarity and the body loses its sensitivity.

There is no invigorating tension associated with premature aging, but there is a definite tightening of the body, beginning with the hips. First, the pelvis opens wide, and the hipbones sink down slightly. This is accompanied by a change in the position of the center of gravity. It is usually located in the center of the body, three fingers' width below the navel. When the pelvis opens and drops, the center of gravity moves to the front of the body. This puts pressure on the pubic bone, which moves forward, and this change of position causes the upper body to move backward. The result is (in an exaggerated rendition) a body in the shape of an S, where the top of the S is the head and the bottom of the S is the top of the thighs and backside. The back tends to be curved and the hips thrust forward.

Unfortunately, few if any people realize the relationship between their change of posture and the decline of their sexual energy. The primary reason is that this posture feels comfortable to the individual. Should he or she try to stand up straight, it would be difficult to maintain that posture. However, because this posture is not gradually acquired as part of the aging process, one feels a little confused about why this should happen. Should confusion persist, it will lead to anxiety as the individual loses confidence in his or her body to correct itself.

People whose bodies assume this shape find it most comfortable to bend forward. This is immediately apparent in the way they sit, which is at the edge of their seats, leaning forward.

Premature aging is almost always accompanied by a feeling of tiredness or fatigue. Thoughts of desire of any kind lose their hard-edge definition and become vague. One can, perhaps, "psyche oneself up" to sexual arousal, but the desire is short-lived and is not accompanied by the necessary physical tension. If one is forced to perform sex through "obligation," it is unsatisfying to both parties.

Should a person experiencing the "fatigue" of premature aging practice *kiryū*, he or she would soon find that the entire body is not fatigued, but only a small part of it, and that qi will collect at that part in order to invigorate it.

Qi Treatment for Premature Aging and for Restoring Sexual Energy

The first thing an individual with waning sexual energy should do is work on himself. This means doing the breathing exercises given at the beginning of the book.

The pelvis has opened, the body has to some extent slumped forward, and both the pelvis and vertebrae have become rigid. Therefore, the individual should lie on his back, and breathe through the spine. If possible, you should do the procedure given on pages 38 to 41, in which you breathe through the top of your head and down the spine. This has the effect of instantly relaxing the mind and the individual vertebrae.

Next, still lying on your back, try sending breath in the form of white vapor from your nose to your genitals and back again. Once your body has relaxed by doing this, inhale through your nose and exhale through your genitals. Specifically, a man will exhale through his testicles, and a woman will exhale through her ovaries (or where her ovaries used to be if she no longer has them).

Next, *kiryū* is an excellent means of combating fatigue and restoring energy to the places that lack it. You will realize that the sensation of fatigue is not truly body wide, but is confined to a specific body part.

TO STIMULATE A WOMAN

Two or three people working on the woman will produce results more quickly than a person working alone.

There are two points that require stimulation: the sides of the bridge of the nose (see Figure 5.1 on page 139) and just below the balls of the feet. The ovaries (see Figure 4.14 on page 95) should be monitored at the same time qi is given, in order to gauge how the treatment is progressing.

With the woman lying on her back, the giver places his thumbs alongside the bridge of her nose and imagines sending qi into her ovaries. Another person standing at the woman's feet will feel the qi flow out of the soles of her feet, just below the ball of each foot. Sitting, he should place the hearts of his hands over this point on each foot, and send qi upward toward the other giver. If a third person is handy, she can place her hands above the ovaries and feel the qi flowing out and upward from the ovaries. If a third person is not available, the woman can do it herself.

The qi will not flow for a while, perhaps as long as two minutes, but soon it will begin to exit the ovaries and flow up toward the ceiling. It will intensify in strength. After two or three minutes, the strength of the qi will begin to wane, and this is the time for both givers to stop sending qi and end on a synchronized exhalation.

The treatment continues below.

TREATING MEN AND WOMEN

1. The receiver lies on his back. The giver stands or sits behind him, and places his palms under the receiver's head, the hearts of his hands resting under the base of the skull (see Figure 5.5 on page 151). Put qi in for two minutes.

2. The receiver turns over onto his stomach. Tap the back of the head lightly with two fingers about fifteen times. This will relax the sacrum.

3. Place the palm of your right hand over the sacrum, and send qi into it for one minute.

4. Place your thumbs alongside L3, and pressing gently but firmly, send qi in for two minutes. Next, place your right thumb directly over L3, and send qi in for two minutes. This vertebra regulates the flexibility of the pelvis. Now do the same to T7. This vertebra stimulates the endocrine system.

5. Finally, place the palm of your right hand over Head Point Number 5, and send qi in for one minute. As you send qi into this point, explain to the receiver that sexual feelings are good and come in many different forms; that these feelings may be channeled into desire for success, fame, creativity, and so on; and that sexual performance is not an issue, but that it is likely to return as various desires return.

6. In cases where the body has slouched forward from the pubic bone and the lower back is weak, the individual should stand and, keeping his knees straight, touch his toes a half dozen times a day. If possible, the individual should attempt to touch his palms to the floor.

Remember: the goal of these treatments is the restoration of sexual energy, not necessarily the restoration of sexual performance. The treatments are meant to remove fatigue and lethargy, and to restore one's interest in life. Sexual desire and sexual performance quite often accompany a return of sexual energy. However, performance is strongly linked to psychology, and this may be beyond the power of qi to influence. Therefore, patience is advised. Once sexual energy returns, it may be channeled at some time back to the sexual act.

CASE HISTORY

Jenny was brought to see me when she was forty-three. She and her husband, Art, wrote screenplays for television and films, and had established a respectable career. Jenny was full of energy—it was she who came up with ideas for new scripts and who got the ideas down quickly on paper while Art contacted agents and managers.

Shortly after concluding a successful screenplay, Jenny seemed to slip into a mild depression. She lost interest in food, in exercise, in getting and spending money, and even in developing new projects. Art assumed she had "postproduction depression" and was very deferential to her feelings and concerned about her welfare.

By the third month, however, he was beginning to lose patience. It was as if desire in all its forms had left her, and she had become apathetic to all of his ideas for fun and excitement, not to mention his hints at romance and sexual advances. They had not had sex since her "depression" began, and she took no interest in him beyond daily civilities. Still, he said nothing until she complained of lower backache, and it was for this that he brought her to see me. He told me nothing except that she had lower backache and seemed mildly depressed.

Her posture indicated premature aging. She said that she had taken to sitting at the edge of the toilet seat when she urinated, and kept her heels off the floor so that she could lean forward. She never used to do it; it just felt more comfortable now. In fact, Art had noticed that her posture, especially her seated posture, had changed from reclining to leaning forward.

She also said that she had not menstruated in four months—from the time her "depression" began—which indicated rigidity of the pelvis. When I checked her pelvis, it was closed tight and was unresponsive to qi.

She had come to see me for lower backache, not for any sex-related matter, and I hesitated to bring it up. However, Art was concerned for her overall welfare, not just her lower back, and I would need his help to work effectively on her. Thus, I decided to be candid, explained the phenomenon of premature aging and its relation to a decline in sexual energy, and concluded by asking Art for his help during the treatment. His response was dramatic.

"Give me back my wife," he exclaimed. "I'll do anything to help."

As neither of them knew anything about qi, a brief introduction was necessary, but through generosity of spirit, Art's qi flowed out strongly and steadily. With me at her head and Art at her feet, we soon had a lot of qi flowing out of her ovaries, and Jenny was amazed at how easily she could feel the changes in flow and temperature with her hands.

We gave qi in this way for five minutes, and then had her turn over. I gave her the standard treatment to restore sexual energy. Art insisted on standing by her side and putting qi into her wherever he could without being in my way.

When the treatment ended, her posture had improved so that sitting at the edge of her seat was no longer comfortable. It felt better to recline. Her lower backache was gone.

After the third treatment, Art phoned me to say, "She's come back to me. Thank you."

After the fourth treatment, Jenny craved to buy a new, large house, indicating the end of premature aging and a return to "normal." The cost of the house, Art admitted, strained them financially, and so they would not be able to afford any more treatments. He apologized for making me a victim of my own success.

CHAPTER 8

Qi and the Ultimate Transition

A Parable

I am not sure why I saved this parable for the final chapter. It is relevant to this book from beginning to end. It was an intuitive act and, from the feeling of qi, the right thing to do.

Sometime around 25 B.C., a young Hindu ascetic found himself perplexed. There were so many different religions and schools of religious thought, each claiming its own superiority in the attainment and exposition of Truth. The young man decided to visit all the various schools of thought and houses of worship, seeking the religious leaders therein, in order to pose the following problem: standing on one leg, the sage must explain the essence of his religion. The young ascetic would offer his allegiance and devotion to whoever passed this test.

He traveled throughout India, Persia, and Hellenized Syria, seeking out famous religious leaders. And to each he posed the problem. Each sage took up the challenge eagerly and with great confidence in his ability to expound the Truth while standing on one leg.

"You see," each sage began, "in the beginning there was this, which led to that, and so on until we come to this, which led us to conceive that . . ."

After a couple of minutes, the leg supporting the sage would begin to tremble, and after another minute, he would fall over before he had even begun to discuss Truth. The Hindu was disappointed, but was determined to visit Rome and beyond if that was what it took to hear the truth.

He was not destined to go that far. In the fifth year of his travels, he arrived in Jerusalem, and was told that a man named Hillel was a great sage with a genius for expounding the Truth. The ascetic went straight to his school and put the problem to him. Hillel listened gravely.

"The essence, eh?" he mused, and then smiling, said that nothing could be easier. Raising his left leg, he said, "Compassion," and lowered the leg.

"But how can you say that? The essence of your religion has got to be more than one word!" exclaimed the young ascetic. "Do you not have a lengthy Bible, and Torah, and Talmud and more? What do they represent?"

"Commentary," replied Hillel, and waved the young man away.

Caretaking of the Terminally Ill and Elderly

This section is meant not only for the caregiver (the person who lifts, carries, wipes, cleans, and feeds), but also for concerned family and friends who give time and attention to the caregiven.

The qi giver must have compassion for the person he is endeavoring to help. This holds true for any situation, but it is especially important to bear this in mind when working with the terminally ill, the dying, and the very old.

Compassion is a powerful frame of mind that maintains its objective integrity. It looks upon objects and circumstances unmoved by impulse or high emotion. It is the supreme form of pity and tenderness.

Sympathy and a wish to do good at any cost are weak emotions that are at the mercy of subjectivity. They internalize an external problem, and frequently lead to wishing to put oneself in another's place, or to take another's pain upon oneself. One frequently has the feeling that one "has been there and felt that," and that one has the ability to deal with another's problem.

It is ear-catching political rhetoric to announce in varying degrees of sincerity, "I feel your pain." The fact of the matter is, the politician neither does nor can feel another's pain. One cannot internalize poverty or child abuse.

On the contrary, you the qi giver are very susceptible to another's pain. A gush of sympathy opens the door to the receiver's qi entering you and bringing its problems with it. A qi giver who sympathizes with a receiver in the middle of an anxiety attack will himself become anxious, even panicky. To try to understand another's stomach pain while giving qi to the stomach will bring that pain into your stomach.

Compassion keeps the mind focused and objective, allowing us to make the right move at the right time. Sympathy negates our objectivity, and clouds our judgment.

On the third day of a recent five-day qi workshop, a participant complained of the sudden onset of a severe headache. One of the other participants exclaimed, "You poor dear. I know just how that feels. Let me give you qi." She raced over and put her hands on the other woman's head, and as fast as thought, the headache entered her and caused her to cry with pain. When I felt her head, the qi was stationary, and just whirled in a small space like a dog chasing its tail. These were the exact same symptoms that the first woman presented. She had unwittingly taken the woman's pain upon herself, and was no longer an effective provider of qi. She would have provided relief and saved herself a headache by remaining dispassionate and acting out of compassion.

A sympathetic qi caregiver says, "I will share that person's pain."

A compassionate qi caregiver says, "I will remove that person's pain."

The need to remain objective and compassionate is applicable to any qi-giving situation. I call this state of mind "dispassionate and compassionate." By "dispassionate" I mean fair, objective, impartial, and level-headed. It is vital to bear these words in mind when caretaking the terminally ill, for it is all too tempting to become sympathetic and try to "save" them. You will simply take their frailties and afflictions upon yourself, and lose your ability to provide them with effective care.

Sympathy for a dying loved one or terminally ill person will result in the diminution of your own powers.

International epidemiological studies of the elderly and their lifestyle have shown that, regardless of country or culture, an older person living with a younger person does not grow young under the influence of the younger person. To the contrary, the younger person "grows old" and assumes the characteristics of the elder.

In the same way, sympathy and a desire to do good at any cost will corrupt your integrity as an effective caretaker. You will come to resemble your charge.

Compassion and a generosity of spirit are the most important elements in caretaking with qi.

Caretakers must first take care of themselves in order to provide effective care.

Some years ago, I was preparing to leave the following day for Japan when I received a call from the personal manager of a rock star. The rock star was suffering lower back spasms and sciatica. His upcoming tour was in jeopardy. Would I drop everything and check him out?

Being the caring person I am, I told the manager that I was busy with my own life, and to just shoot him full of painkillers until I returned. Anyway, he probably had enough money that canceling a tour wouldn't matter.

"Of course it wouldn't hurt him financially," his manager replied, "but think of all the people who depend on him. The guys in his band and their wives and children. Then the technicians and roadies. How about the people who sell souvenirs? They have families to support. How about the kids who sell soft drinks at the concerts? They're probably supporting their parents or making money for college. Don't you realize how many people will be adversely affected if he is unable to tour?"

The caregiver is like that rock star. Without your own good health and sound judgment, those who depend on you will be adversely affected. Your state of mind and body must come before that of your charge(s).

Do not fall into the trap of "caretaker captivity."

Do not let sympathy or routine enslave you to your charge. For many caregiven, particularly the very old, their loss of physical independence arouses in them the desire to have some sort of sway over another person. They will play upon a caregiver's sympathy or sense of duty to bend that person to their will. This is how they exercise their qi. To cooperate with the caregiver would seem like capitulation and resignation to their loss of independence; while to the contrary, resistance and conflict energize the caregiven and restore to them a measure of (emotional) independence.

Among the hallmarks of caretaker captivity are an increasing reluctance to delegate authority or responsibility, and an assumption that everyone else in the caretaking enterprise is negligent and incompetent. This means repeated phone calls to the doctor's office, nurses' station, medical-equipment provider, nursing home staff, and so on. This means worry that the caregiven's diet is not being seen to, or that the care is inadequate even though the nursing staff has just been instructed exactly what to do.

This caretaker's captivity keeps one's qi from flowing steadily throughout the body. It tends to collect in the head, and so produces repetitive, anxious, and negative thoughts. It will lead to loss of sleep and loss of appetite. More and more, you come to resemble your charge.

As caregiver, you must have time for yourself. You must have the freedom to enjoy yourself. You must be able to exercise and maintain your health. You must keep regular mealtimes and eat what you like in a relaxed frame of mind. You must keep a healthy perspective of your abilities and limitations: specifically, what you can provide your charge and what is beyond your power to provide. You may compromise with the caregiven, but you must not capitulate to what you consider to be bad behavior. And finally, you must feel that, by caregiving with qi, you are actively participating in the health and welfare of your charge. This last article is particularly important.

Caregiving involves physical labor, much of it dirty and unrewarding. It is sad if the caregiver or family member becomes a captive to that role and that role alone without being able to participate in the health of their charge. Most caregivers are concerned bystanders who feel powerless to do anything but watch and wait as physicians, technicians, and therapists play the dominant health-care role in the lives of their charges.

By means of the techniques given in this book, the caregiver can become an active and health-effective participant in the life of her charge.

Giving qi to the caregiven will alleviate pain, lessen the side effects of drugs, improve appetite, stimulate alertness, and provide physical and spiritual comfort.

The means to give qi to these ends are all listed in this book.

Remember: when giving qi to those over age eighty, the treatment should be short and intense. It is better to give two short treatments than one long treatment. It is for the caregiver to adapt his position to provide maximum comfort to the care-given. Many ill and elderly are unable to sit or turn over. Be resourceful in how you give qi.

1. Giving qi locally will alleviate pain. Giving qi to the solar plexus will create a feeling of comfort and warmth (see Figure 4.17 on page 101), as will holding the right arm (see Figure 2.15 on page 49).

2. Giving qi to Head Point Number 5 will promote sleep (pages 119–120), as will giving qi to the heart of the right hand (page 119). Giving qi to Head Points Number 2 will promote alertness and health of nerves and organs. It will also improve the appetite and digestion.

3. Giving qi to the liver will promote body cleansing. Giving qi to the lymph glands under the armpits will also stimulate body cleansing (see Figure 5.4 on page 139).

4. Look for a head groove between Head Point Numbers 3 and 5, and if it is present, give direct qi to improve appetite and to overcome trauma.

5. Finally, the very act of hands-on qi giving provides an intimate bond between care-giver and caregiven. It is not just physical comfort, but also emotional succor. Providing and receiving hands-on qi care is the physical manifestation of the mind/body union of both parties.

If you are not sure what kind of treatment to provide, I strongly recommend giving qi while you are under the influence of *kiryū*. Once you have attained a facility with *kiryū*, your hands will wander over the caregiven's body, locating impediments to the flow of qi. Once your hands have located these spots, they will remain there giving qi until the obstacle (usually tension) has been removed. They will then move on to the next spot.

The physical sensation of receiving qi in this way is very pleasurable to the caregiven, and the results are no less effective than giving qi more systematically. Best of all, the caregiver sees to her own health even as she sees to the health of her charge.

Final Guidance

The ideal place to participate in the final passage of a loved one is a homey environment—at home itself, in a hospice, in a nursing home, or in an assisted-care facility. The atmosphere should be tranquil, so that each person can be full of her own thoughts and memories, and sensitive to the qi moving through the loved one. The deeper the thought, the more loving the intention, the richer and fuller the qi will be.

If possible, there should be at least three people at the deathbed giving qi: one for the Achilles tendons, one for the neck and solar plexus, and one for the liver. A fourth person will cover the heart of the hand with the heart of her own hand, and a fifth person will take the other hand.

However, this ideal is not always attainable. **One person alone, seated at the right side of the caregiven—giving qi with the left hand beneath the neck, the right hand on the solar plexus—is enough to guide the loved one through the final passage.**

In the case of more than one person, the qi givers should be seated comfortably. Each person should have a word to say about the loved one—a fond memory or loving sentiment. Then, synchronizing your breaths, send qi into the body as you exhale simultaneously. Having done this, you may breathe at your own pace. There is no need to synchronize your breaths again until you decide to end the procedure.

The person(s) at the Achilles tendons and the person at the solar plexus should send qi back and forth. At first, you will not feel one another's qi coming into your hands. After a minute or two, you will feel the other's qi flowing in strongly and steadily, and you may be assured that there is no blockage or impediment to qi in the body.

The person at the liver will be able to monitor the flow of qi between all the parties as well as the loved one's response.

The more you think fondly about the person to whom you are giving qi, the stronger the qi will flow.

Do not think that you are going to postpone the final moment or produce a miraculous recovery.

In fact, do not think anything but affectionate thoughts for the person whom you are touching. Any thoughts of "doing something" to stave off the final moment will be counterproductive and will interfere with the steady flow of qi through the person's body. In a sense, you have to actively acquiesce to the other's fate. Your compassion and sorrow will not in any way be diminished by this. Quite the opposite: you will have a firm bond with the person whom you are guiding, and your feelings will be the more profound for that.

A REMARKABLE EXPERIENCE

I have been involved with qi medicine as student and teacher for more than twenty years. During that time I have heard of, witnessed, and participated in any number of "inexplicable remissions," "miracle cures," and "extraordinary events." It took me about ten years to come to the conclusion that this is the way qi works, and that the miracle is the human body, not the healing technique. The technique is, to put it in an Irish way, very simple if you know how. The body's resilience and flexibility is what is truly astonishing. The following story is, to me, one of *the* most remarkable qi events I have ever witnessed, as well as a testament to the body's glorious flexibility.

I had heard "incredible" tales about giving qi to the dying and was finally privileged to experience it.

My Japanese friend, Ono, is very skilled at qi healing, and has introduced the qi way of life and health to his whole family, and that includes his elderly parents and parents-in-law. They do *kiryū* on a regular basis, either alone or in combination of partners. The entire family enjoys good health.

When Ono's father turned ninety, the family held a celebration, and I, too, was invited. The father, though feeble, showed every sign of good health. Three months later, Ono phoned me mid-morning to say that his father had suffered a stroke three days after the party, and was not expected to survive much longer. He was resting at home and was free of pain. The entire family had gathered round him to give qi. Would I like to come over and help guide him through the final passage? Of course, I would be honored, I replied, and went over straightaway.

Ono, his wife, and his two children were giving qi to the old man. Each child held a hand over one Achilles tendon, his wife was giving qi to his liver, and Ono was cradling his father's neck with his left hand and giving qi to the solar plexus with his right. I was invited to place my hand over the heart of Ono's father's left hand. We synchronized our breaths to begin giving qi, and then breathed at our own pace, giving qi all the while.

The old man's body was very warm, though his brain seemed lifeless. I could feel the family's qi passing through my hand, and I could feel that there was an increase in the intensity of the qi as it came from the family and from the old man himself.

And then, I was summoned by cell phone to respond to a mini-crisis. When I returned an hour later, the old man was dead. The four family members had not moved and were continuing to give qi.

"Too bad," Ono said, "you missed the explosion of qi. He went off with a bang about half an hour ago."

Ono's mother appeared about fifteen minutes later, and felt her late husband's forehead. It was still warm and moist. He did not seem dead. She spoke to him calmly as if he were going to climb off the table any second. Then she left the room to call the funeral home.

We continued giving qi to the body for another thirty minutes. Now, here comes the incredible part.

The body stayed warm for the rest of the afternoon, and rigor mortis (rigidity of the corpse) still had not begun when I left the house five hours later. Rigor mortis begins at the face and moves downward, frequently beginning as soon as ten minutes after death. Six hours had passed, and rigor mortis was not at all apparent. The old man's body was as warm and as flexible as that of a living person. I had heard about this phenomenon in qi circles, but never expected to witness or experience it for myself.

I later asked Ono if rigor mortis had set in. He replied, "Yes, but quite later. None of us was very aware of time. It was probably the middle of the evening when someone from the funeral home said that the body was growing rigid. Isn't it strange?"

Sublimed Qi

I have been half in love with easeful Death.

—JOHN KEATS

The undiscovered country, from whose bourn No traveller returns.

—SHAKESPEARE

You can provide physical relief and spiritual comfort to the caregiven as shown above. But do not fall into the error of conceiving of death as an enemy, especially an enemy with a will of its own. It is to the benefit of neither the caregiver nor caregiven to slip into Dylan Thomas's state of mind when he pleaded with his father, in the poem "Do Not Go Gentle into That Good Night":

> *Old age should burn and rave at close of day,*
> *Rage, rage against the dying of the light.*

These are the words of a young healthy man, not the sentiments of an elderly man; certainly not those of an elderly man inching his way toward death. For many, if not most of the dying, Keats's words are more relevant and beneficial to caregiver and caregiven alike. Death is often the most healthy alternative left to the dying, and it can seem very tempting indeed to one who is suffering or who has lost the capacity for any enjoyment and satisfaction.

Kayoko Matsuura died at the age of eighty-four, and the manner of her death was as startling to me as her outlook on life. It was from her that I learned that qi is sublimed—meaning purified—at the moment of death. It departs from the organism to the purity of its own existence.

She suffered a stroke and, through sheer force of will, brought herself back to a semblance of health. She was bedridden. She could not walk or use her hands well, but she could speak and think clearly. She did *kiryū* in the only way that was left her: she shouted at the top of her lungs over and over until her entire body vibrated and her breath deepened from a shout to a roar.

The last time I saw her she confided in me that she had decided to die. She had spent her life actively giving qi and helping people. Now she was confined to a meager margin of existence. Life was weakness; death was strength. Living was passive; dying was active. She was going to exercise her qi in the only positive way left her, by dying.

I did not understand her. I thought, perhaps, she was suffering some sort of dementia brought on by the stroke. At university, I had read Zen texts in which the ancient patriarchs sought eccentric ways to die. One died standing on his head, another shouted and dropped dead, another just stood still until he died. To me, these were anecdotes of enlightened zanies that could not be confirmed or denied. How could someone decide to die? And more, how could anyone as feeble as she put that determination into action?

We said our good-byes. She clamped her jaws shut and armored herself in qi. Her jaws could not be pried open, and her body rejected all attempts at intravenous intervention. She died two days after our final farewell.

And now comes, perhaps, the best reason for practicing qi with those you love, admire, and wish never to leave.

The event occurred about eighteen months after my last qi treatment from Kayoko Matsuura. I was looking for a new practitioner and teacher to replace her, and was recommended to a man who had a large practice and a formidable reputation. He put his hands on my head, and then on the base of my spine. After five minutes, he said, "You have a sharp, eccentric sort of qi. It reminds me very much of a practitioner I used to know, but haven't seen for a few years. Her name was Kayoko Matsuura, and she had the sort of qi that once experienced is never forgotten. Have you ever received qi from her?"

Her qi lives on in me, and thus she lives on in me. Not as a memory, but as a palpable force.

Earlier I wrote that when I do my qi warm-ups, I think of people, living and dead, whom I admire and whose approval I seek. I dedicate the good I will do that day to a certain person. I call this "Dedicated Qi."

When I dedicate my qi to someone whose qi I know, and whose qi I have often felt, I can feel their qi entering me from some external abode. I feel a fusion of my qi and their qi into a much larger, more potent qi than I could possibly create by myself.

I *feel* Kayoko Matsuura's presence when I dedicate my qi to her. I can connect in a physical way with old teachers, friends, and family whenever I choose.

I do not receive messages from "the other side," and I am not privy to the secrets of the universe via Kahlewa, ancient warrior lounge-queen. The spirit of J. P. Morgan does not provide me with stock tips. What I experience is the physical presence of familiar qi from friends and loved ones. Each qi has its own "signature." I can read the signature and feel assured that I have access to that person's qi.

Your qi therefore becomes a repository of the lives of all those who have (literally and figuratively) touched you.

Our qi does not wane with illness or old age. It maintains its integrity until the final moment of life. What does change is our biorhythm. The duration of ebb tide becomes longer, and flood tide becomes brief, but intense. This accounts for sudden remissions or bursts of energy in the dying. The qi has returned to the center of the body, to the flood tide position, and the organism is stimulated to activity. After the energy surge, the tide ebbs and lingers for another long interval.

And at the final moment of life, all of the qi collects in the center of the body, and there is an efflorescence or explosion of qi—thus, the numerous eyewitness accounts of auras or bursts of light emitted from the dying at the moment of death. I have been present at only a few peaceful deaths, but I have heard from other qi practitioners that death, like birth, always occurs at flood tide (or produces the flood tide), and then all is silence. Though the organism is still active (hair and nails still grow, and organs can still be harvested for transplant), qi has departed, and the organism is now pronounced lifeless.

A FAMILY STORY

My grandmother Celia was a very hardheaded woman. No one could possibly sell her snake oil or shares in a beefsteak mine. Yet this I'll-believe-it-when-I-see-it grandmother witnessed the ultimate qi event, and became an instant convert to the existence of qi.

Her husband, Bill, had been unconscious for more than two years. He had been pronounced a "healthy vegetable," meaning his physiology was strong though he existed in unconsciousness. He had a ravenous appetite, but did not know what he ate.

As he approached his ninetieth birthday, his vital signs began to fail. Celia began a bedside deathwatch. Given his deathlike condition, it seemed almost impossible to know if he had slipped away into death or if he still had an ounce of life in him.

Suddenly, he opened his eyes and stared intelligently at his wife. "His eyes," she said later, "were bright blue and penetrating."

He smiled and called her by name as if he had just awoken from a catnap. His voice was firm and resonant. Then he closed his eyes, and "shining blue-gray energy rose out of his body, hovered for a moment, and then vanished."

When my grandmother felt him, he was dead.

Subsequent to this experience, my grandmother held definite, positive views on the subject of the conservation of energy. She believed in a universal pool of qi. She saw for herself that her husband had been transmuted to go . . . It didn't matter where, but that he had been transmuted and then vanished could not be disputed.

The family was astonished by *her* subsequent transformation. She had been transmuted from a no-nonsense old woman who talked about people "kicking the bucket" to a believer in death as a purifying and mystical event. Witnessing the efflorescence of her husband's qi was one of the great events of her life.

How I Would Like to Die

A number of qi practitioners gather at irregular intervals in Tokyo and swap stories, discuss interesting or unusual cases, report on new techniques and "discoveries," and share personal histories of birth and death. The following story was told at such a gathering by a middle-aged woman. I was touched by the story and by the sentiment with which she conveyed the story's events. When I returned home from the meeting, I transcribed her story as faithfully as memory allowed.

"My mother died of extreme old age. She was ninety-five years and one month old. She had been introduced to qi more than forty years before, and from the age of sixty-four, she began practicing qi on friends and family. Of course, she did *kiryū* daily until she was no longer able.

"She died from deterioration of mind and body. She always hoped she would go quickly and quietly, and that is how she went. Her senility became apparent from age ninety. From that time she had as many lucid days as senile days, and on her lucid days, she continued to practice qi. However, from age ninety-one, her number of lucid days declined, and she began to forget familiar names and faces, even family members, though not when she was face-to-face with us.

"From age ninety-one she began sleeping more and eating less. She needed to lie down from time to time. These signs of deterioration were so obvious that we were sure she would soon die. Death became a houseguest. We always had our radar pointed in Mother's direction, and were sensitive to react to changes in her state of alertness and physical strength. She spent a lot of time in bed giving herself qi. When I would give her qi, she would always move my hand from where I had placed it, and replace it on a different part of her body. And it was always the right place. I mean, the qi flowed into that point smoothly. She particularly enjoyed receiving qi to her head.

"From age ninety-three she became willful and refused to be told what to do. She would try to walk out of the house, even in the middle of winter. Her willfulness became a nightmare when she became incontinent. She would fight against any help, and would not use a diaper until the very last moment. It was always touch and go if she would get the diaper on in time. Of course she frequently miscalculated, and then there was a real mess to clean up.

"She was cheerful to our two girls, and loved being asked to give them qi. She had known them since the womb, and they are both 'imprinted' with her qi. They responded well to her qi, and giving them qi never failed to energize her.

"Her final deterioration came a month before her death. She grew oblivious to toileting, and, like a baby, would lie around in diapers, saying nothing when she soiled herself.

"However, even with this deterioration, she sat with us at dinner each evening. She seemed lucid. She ate almost nothing, but would smile at me and the girls with her lips forming the shape of a kiss. Then she'd say, 'Let's all go there,' and smile radiantly. The gentle radiance of her smile is the most memorable feature of her life for me.

"One day, she seemed changed. I can't quite explain how, but there was something about her that frightened me. I placed my hand on her to give qi, but she did not move it as she usually did. I put the heart of my hand on her solar plexus. The space between the ribs seemed to be filled with a wooden plank. Her solar plexus was impenetrable. Qi would not go in, not a drop. I became frantic and started searching her body for an opening that would receive qi, but after a moment, I felt as if I was violating her body by searching all over for it. Her body seemed to have no moisture. I removed my hand and left her to sleep.

"I asked her physician to come to the house the next day. He listened to her chest and looked into her eyes. He was very professional and very gentle. He said, 'She's not going to last much longer. Now is not the time to do anything that will give her pain. When she passes away, relax, note the time, and phone me when you feel composed.'

"From that night, Mother slept between me and my eldest daughter. She wanted her hand held as she slept, and we took turns.

"Two days later, Mother was sitting with us at dinner. She had no interest in food, but asked me to feel the back of her head. It was very cold. The next morning, while she was asleep, I felt for the 'plank' around her solar plexus, and it had become lumpy. I mean physically bumpy and lumpy. I had no idea what the lumps were or what they meant.

"When I think about these final days, I mean the last week of her life, what strikes me as extraordinary was how routine and ordinary family life was. It was as if there was no dying woman in the house. The family was calm, and home life was peaceful.

"The end came a week after the physician's visit. It was Christmas evening. Mother began making small sounds, and I sat by her side, giving qi to the back of her head and solar plexus. My younger daughter was crying softly. She said, 'Thank you for everything, Grandma.' At that moment, the plank disappeared from Mother's solar plexus, and her body relaxed. Her face became tranquil and all of her wrinkles vanished. Her complexion grew rosy and almost transparent. I could not believe my eyes.

"'Did you see that?' I asked the girls. Both of them nodded.

"The elder girl said, 'You're not dead yet, Grandma, you can still give me qi.'

"Mother reached out and took her hand between her thumb and forefinger, looked deeply at the girl, and began giving qi. 'Death will keep us together,' she said in a whisper.

"Her breath became irregular. Suddenly, my daughter shouted and jumped back as if she had received an electric shock. Mother was dead. Her qi had exploded out of her and into my daughter. Her passing was tranquil and gentle.

"I wondered then and wonder now, where did the wrinkles go? Why did her skin turn transparent? She was absolutely beautiful. She had never ever been so beautiful, and she remained so until the funeral.

"To be honest, I'm lonely without her. But I am forever grateful at the wonder she showed me. There are limits to life; she revealed to me what we can do within those limits. And I learned from experience that even at the instant of death, our will and feelings and qi are as active as they were at the moment of birth. Which leads me to wonder if we do have an end . . . ?"

How I Try to Live

Working with qi for more than twenty years has not brought me any closer to apprehending the meaning of life. It has not provided me with a philosophy of guidance and comfort. What it has done is validate the wisdom of William Blake when he wrote that "Exuberance is Beauty." The exuberance obtained from the energy of qi, the exuberance that informs our best actions, the exuberance that comes of knowing that we are not living in a fragmented universe, but one that is unified by qi—all of this exuberance is, indeed, very beautiful.

I would like to close this chapter and this book on a note of exuberance. It is a Japanese poem (my translation) that provides me all the guidance and comfort for which I have ever yearned.

> *If you seek death,*
> *Then die! If life,*
> *Live on!*
> *But, oh! What joy*
> *Just to have been born*
> *In this world.*

—TANAKA SHOZO (1841–1913)

There are seven cervical, twelve thoracic, and five lumbar vertebrae. This is a guide to the signposts leading to about half of all the vertebrae.

Cervical Vertebra 2
(*C2*)—Located at the base of the skull.

Cervical Vertebra 3
(*C3*)—In line with the lower edge of the ear-lobes.

Cervical Vertebra 7
(*C7*)—This is the largest cervical vertebra. It protrudes when you bend your neck forward. It is the southern-most vertebra to turn when the head turns.

Thoracic Vertebra 1
(*T1*)—The next in line after C7. It is the first vertebra that does not turn when the head turns.

Thoracic Vertebra 5
(*T5*)—This vertebra frequently protrudes.

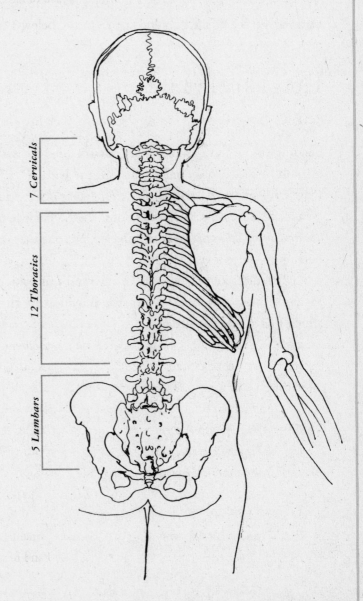

7 Cervicals

12 Thoracics

5 Lumbars

Thoracic Vertebra 6 (T6)—Located directly behind the solar plexus.

Thoracic Vertebra 7 (T7)—Located in line with the lower edge of the scapula.

Thoracic Vertebra 11 (T11)—Located in the middle of the back where most women fasten their bra.

Thoracic Vertebra 12 (T12)—The last vertebra to have a rib attached to it.

Lumbar Vertebra 1 (L1)—About two inches below T11, and much larger than the thoracic vertebrae. *L2 - related to the function of the intestines cleanses the brain and nervous system*

Lumbar Vertebra 3 (L3)—Located directly behind the navel, and corresponds to the waistline. *regulates the movement of the pelvis*

Lumbar Vertebra 4 (L4)—This vertebra lies in line with the top edge of the pelvis. Standing, place your thumbs at the top of your pelvis, and trace a straight line to your spine. You will land on L4. This can also be done on a receiver lying facedown. *related to the reproductive system, especially its cleansing*

Sacrum—Extends from below L5 to the top of the crack between the buttocks. It consists of five fused bones, counted (from the top) as S1 through S5.

Coccyx—Just below the sacrum.

A WORD ABOUT VERTEBRAE: The vertebrae are bones. The bones themselves do not become tense or rigid or any of the other descriptive words used in this text. Vertebrae are moved by muscles running alongside them, and these muscles become tense and rigid. Tension inhibits the natural movement of the vertebrae, contracts the distance between vertebrae, and, in extreme cases, actually causes the vertebrae to become frozen in a fixed, unmoving position. In short, tension causes a loss of flexibility.

Individual vertebrae can move in eight directions: up, down, left, right, forward (sink), backward (protrude), twist left, and twist right.

The spinal cord is like a hollow conduit with nerves running out of it to organs, regulating the function of these organs. When tension or injury causes one or more vertebrae to lose flexibility or to come out of alignment, the result is a loss of function in the corresponding organ.

When I talk about sending qi into vertebrae to relax the vertebrae and restore flexibility, I mean stimulating the nerves to move and relax the adjoining muscles, which releases the vertebrae from their frozen position and allows them to return to alignment and flexibility.

Vertebrae function individually, as groups, and in combinations. Broadly speaking, the related organs and functions of the vertebrae are given below.

T1–T4—These four vertebrae are related to the brain, the respiratory system, and the heart. They are directly connected to sleep.

T5–T8—These four vertebrae are related to digestion. T6 is directly linked to the stomach.

T9–T12—These four vertebrae are all related to body cleansing, including the kidneys, skin, liver, and bladder.

The five lumbar vertebrae are all related to body cleansing.

L1—Cleanses the brain and nervous system.

L2—Cleanses the intestines.

L3—Cleanses the urinary tract.

L4—Cleanses the reproductive organs.

L5—Cleanses the lungs and respiratory system.

A Handy Guide to the Head

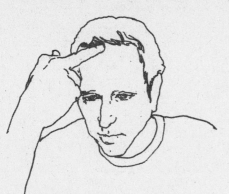

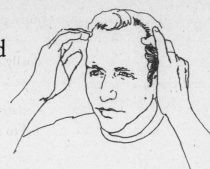

Head Points 2
Located above temples at both sides of head. There is usually a groove or "trench" to indicate the points.

Head Point 1
Located in center of forehead at hairline.

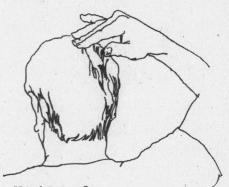

Head Point 3
Located on the   *related to gastric function*
crown of the head.

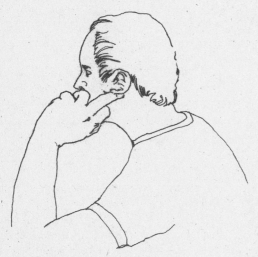

Head Points 4
Located just behind the ear-lobes at the jawline. There is a "dimple" or indentation at these points.

Head Point 5   *related to sleep*
Located on the back and center of the head. It can be found by tracing a line from the top of the eyebrow to the back center of the head. This point is a flat spot the size of a small coin.

Index

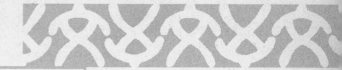

Abdomen, lower, 83
Achilles tendons, 119, 122–23,
    150–51, 172, 202
Adaptation, 6
Adaptive power of body, 53–58
Allopathic medicine, 7
Ankles, 151
Antibiotics, 88
Anxiety, 117
Artificial body parts, 62–63
Asthma, 117, 174
Autonomic nervous system, 60–63
Autumnal changes, 109–110

Baby palace, 128–30
Back, small of, 29
Back pain, lower, 102–5
Balance, 59–60
Biorhythms, 113–15
    case history, 115–16
Blake, William, 45, 211
Body cleansing, 85–86
    case histories, 88, 91–92
    intestines, 88–90
    liver, 89, 91
    menstruation, 93–96
    for pregnant woman, 139–41
    skin, 92–93
    urinary tract, 86–88

Bones, 97–99
Breath, 81–82
    connection between hands and lower
        spine, 28–31
    of God, 14
    powerful circularity of, 31
    quality of and sleep, 116
    visualizing, 25–28

C1 vertebra, 137
C2 vertebra, 99–100, 117, 137, 145,
    212
C3 vertebra, 212
C7 vertebra, 137, 212
Caretaker captivity, 199–200
Caretaking of terminally ill/elderly,
    197–202
Case histories:
    asking baby to tell you its sex,
        157–58
    biorhythms, 115–16
    body cleansing, 88
    ear infections, 174–76
    elderly, 183–85
    newborns, 171
    of pelvis closing after childbirth, 166
    pregnancy, 96–97
    relaxation for infants, toddlers,
        young children, 172–73

sacral pain, 107–8
sexual energy restoration, 193–95
sleep disorders, 124–25
stomach disorders, 84–85
Cervical vertebrae, 137–38
Chekhov, Anton, 59
Childbirth, 162–64. *See also*
        Postpartum period; Pregnancy
Children and qi, 167–69
    case histories, 172–76
    infants, toddlers, young children,
        172–77
    newborns, 169–71
Coccyx, 119, 121–22, 213
Compassion, 197–99

Death and dying, 196–211
Dedicated qi, 206
Digestion, 77–79

Ear infections, 173–74
    case history, 174–76
Early-spring changes, 111
Early-summer changes, 112–13
Eastern medicine, 13
Ebb tide, 113–14
Elderly, 177–81
    caretaking for, 197–202
    case histories, 183–85

Elderly (cont.)
   qi treatments for, 181–82
   Emotional trauma, 78–79
   digestive effects of, 81–83
   Extrapyramidal motor system,
      60–63

Face, 138–40
Feet, 151
Fetus, 134–36, 143
Final passage, 202–4
First trimester, 132. See also
      Childbirth; Pregnancy
   child-rearing awareness, 133–34
   morning sickness during, 143–45
   qi treatment for mother, 137–41
   transmitting qi to fetus, 134–36
   walking during, 141–42
Flexibility, loss of, 177–78
Flood tide, 113–14
Fluid release, 62
Fourth point, 45
Freud, Sigmund, 98

Generosity of spirit, 44–45
Genesis, 14

Hands, 79–80
Hands-on qi, 201
Head, 81, 119–20, 151
   guide to, 215
Head groove, 83, 201
Head Point Number 1, 120
Head Point Number 3, 78, 82, 174
Head Point Number 5, 78, 117, 119–
      20, 145, 170, 173–74, 201
Head Points Number 2, 66–67
Head Points Number 4, 98–99, 140
Health, 5–6
   and qi, 18–21
Healthy energy, 11–12
Heart, 182
Heart of the hand, 119
Heller, Joseph, 16
Hiatal hernia, 81
Hillel, 197
Hypothalamus, 136, 147

Illness, 16–18
Infants, 172–77
Intention, 45
Intestines, 88–90
Ionized water, 89

Johnson, Samuel, 77

Kanji, 1–4, 13
Keats, John, 205
Kidneys, 140
Kiryu, 60–65, 201
   paired, 66–68
   solitary, 68–72
   tales of, 73–74

L1 vertebra, 92, 103, 161, 213–14
L2 vertebra, 88–89, 138, 214
L3 vertebra, 29, 31, 86, 96, 103–5,
      137–38, 161, 165, 213–14
L4 vertebra, 29, 31, 96, 138, 151–52,
      165, 213–14
L5 vertebra, 105, 138, 145, 165, 214
Language development, 167
Left foot, 81
Left leg, 81
Liquor, 92
Liver, 82–83, 89, 91, 119, 122–24,
      144, 171, 173, 201–2
   case history, 91–92
Loss of flexibility, 177–78
Lower abdomen, 83
Lower back pain, 102–5
Lumbar vertebrae, 137–38
Lungs, 182
   developing, 173–75
Lymph glands, 141

Matsuura, Kayoko, 3–5, 63–65, 115,
      124–25, 205–7
Meconium, 169–70
Menstruation, 93–96
Mind/body connection, 78
Mind/body relaxation, 23–24,
      38–41
Miscarriage, 133
Morning sickness, 143–44
   treating, 144–45
Movement, 60
   uninhibited, 61
Mucus, 62
Muscles, 97–99
   treatment for aches and pains,
      99–107

Neck, 202
Neck ache, 99–100
Neck base, 100
Nerve receptors, 97

Newborns, 169–71
Night sweats, 92–93

Ovaries, 93–96, 165
Ovulation, 93

Paired technique:
   for accessing qi, 32–33
   for concentrating and transmitting
      qi, 33–38
Parotid (salivary) glands, 140
Pelvis:
   case history, 166
   in children, 176–77
   closing after childbirth, 164–65
Pets and qi, 41–44
Postpartum period, 164–66
Potatoes, 143
Pregnancy, 126–28. See also Childbirth;
      Postpartum period
   case history, 96–97
   first trimester, 132–45
   and qi, 130–31
   second trimester, 145–58
   third trimester, 159–62
   womb as baby palace, 128–30
Pregnancy rhinitis, 148
Premature aging, 190–91
   qi treatment for, 191–93
Pre-winter changes, 110–11
Pulmonary system, 116–17
Pulse, 114

Qi. See also Qi energy; Qi treatment
   accessing
      advanced procedure, 31
      basic procedure, 24–28
      intermediate procedure, 28–31
      paired technique, 32–33
   applying, 45–46
   breath of God, 14
   and children, 167–69
   concentrating, 33
   and elderly, 177–81
   and generosity of spirit, 44–45
   and health, 18–21
   kanji for, 1–4, 13
   and kiryū, 60–72
   and pets, 41–44
   and pregnant woman, 130–31
   stress and flow of, 58–59
   and terminally ill/elderly,
      196–211

transmitting
    benefits to, 52–53
    to fetus, 134–36
    paired practice, 33–38
    trying too hard with, 50–51
    warming up for, 22–24
Qi energy, 14–16
Qi treatment:
    for constipation, 89–90
    for elderly, 181–82
    for liver function, 91
    for muscle aches and pain,
        99–107
    for muscle tension, 98–99
    for ovaries, 94–96
    for pregnant mother
        in first trimester, 137–41
        in second trimester, 150–52
        in third trimester, 161
    for premature aging, 191–93
    for skin cleansing, 92–93
    for sleep disorders, 119–24
    for stomach disorders, 79–83
    for terminally ill/elderly, 200–204
    for urinary tract, 86–88
Quality of life, 6

Receiver:
    feedback from, 36
    relaxing, 47–49
Relaxation, 46–49, 109
    for infants, toddlers, young children,
        172–73
Rib cage, 81, 121–23
    determining length of, 118

Sacrum, 152, 213
    pain of, 105–7
    case history, 107–8
Seasonal change, 57–58, 108–9
    autumn, 109–10
    early-spring, 111
    early-summer, 112–13
    pre-winter, 110–11
    spring, 111–12
    summer, 113
    winter, 111
Second trimester, 145–46. See also
        Childbirth; Pregnancy
    the baby rises, 152–53
    case history, 157–58

education and discipline in utero,
        153–57
    how is the mother doing?, 148–49
    mother taking stock of her condi-
        tion, 147–48
    qi treatment for mother, 150–52
    sex during, 146–47
    talking out loud to your child,
        149–50
Seiza, 47
Self-maintenance, 52
Sengai, 177–78
Sexual energy, 186–91
    case history, 193–95
    qi treatment for restoring, 191–93
Shakespeare, William, 22, 205
Shoulder, 102
Shoulder blades, 102
Shozo, Tanaka, 211
Skin, 92–93
Sleep disorders, 116–19
    case history, 124–25
    treatment for, 119–24
Small of back, 29
Solar plexus, 100, 201–2
Spindles, 97
Spine:
    guide to, 212–14
    relaxation of, 38–40, 59
Spring changes, 111–12
Stiff shoulders/arms, 100–102
Stomach, 182
Stomach disorders:
    case histories, 84–85
    digestive effects of emotional
        trauma, 81–83
    hiatal hernia, 81
    weak or upset stomach, 79–81
Stress, and flow of qi, 58–59
Sugar, 92
Summer changes, 113
Sympathy, 197–99

T1 vertebra, 118, 120, 122, 173–74,
        212, 214
T2 vertebra, 118, 120, 122, 173–74,
        214
T3 vertebra, 118, 120, 122, 173–74,
        214
T4 vertebra, 118, 120, 122, 173–74,
        214

T5 vertebra, 212, 214
T6 vertebra, 79, 82, 111, 213–14
T7 vertebra, 213–14
T8 vertebra, 214
T9 vertebra, 214
T10 vertebra, 214
T11 vertebra, 86, 110, 140,
        213–14
T12 vertebra, 213–14
Talking internally, 35
Tanden, 67
Tears, 62
Tension, 59, 62, 98–99, 109
Terminally ill, 197–202
Third trimester. See also Childbirth;
        Pregnancy
    education and discipline in utero,
        161–62
    getting the show on the road,
        159–60
    qi treatment for mother, 161
Thomas, Dylan, 205
Tides, 113–14
Toddlers, 172–77
Toxins, 143
Tranquil point, 45
Trauma, emotional, 78–79
Treatment. See Qi treatment

Upper arm hold, 49–50
Urinary tract, 86–88, 144

Vertebrae, 212–14. See also individual
        vertebrae
Vocalized sounds, 62

Waist, 141
Walking, 141–42
Watabe, Takeski, 2, 184
Weak/upset stomach, 79–81
Well-being, 5
Western medicine, 7, 17
Whiplash, 79
White vapor, 25–28
Winter changes, 111
Womb, 128–30

Yawning, 61–62
Young children, 172–77